CRASH COURSE
Imaging

D1528966

Other titles in the Crash Course series

There are 23 books in the Crash Course series in two ranges: Basic Science and Clinical. Each book follows the same format, with concise text, clear illustrations and helpful learning features including access to online USMLE test questions.

Basic Science titles
Pathology
Nervous System
Renal and Urinary Systems
Gastrointestinal System
Respiratory System
Endocrine and Reproductive Systems
Metabolism and Nutrition
Pharmacology
Immunology
Musculoskeletal System
Cardiovascular System
Cell Biology and Genetics
Anatomy

Clinical titles
Surgery
Cardiology
History and Examination
Internal Medicine
Neurology
Gastroenterology
OBGYN
Psychiatry
Pediatrics

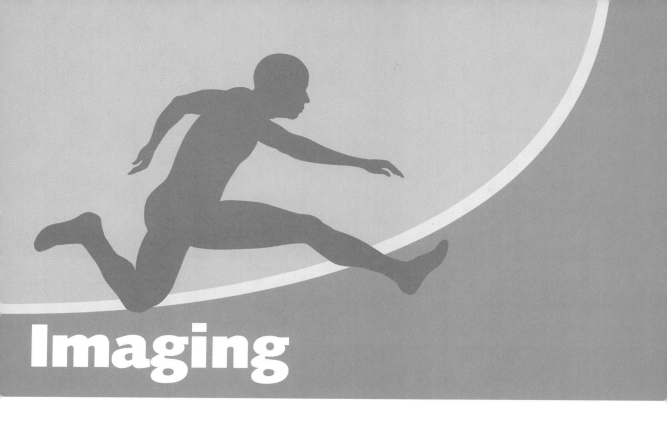

Imaging

Deborah ter Meulen, MD
Division of Breast Imaging
Department of Radiology
Massachusetts General Hospital
Boston, Massachusetts

UK edition authors
Barry Kelly and Ian C. Bickle

UK series editor
Daniel Horton-Szar

MOSBY

ELSEVIER

1600 John F. Kennedy Blvd.
Suite 1800
Philadelphia, PA 19103-2899

CRASH COURSE: IMAGING   ISBN-13: 978-0-323-05338-9
Copyright © 2008 by Mosby, Inc., an affiliate of Elsevier Inc.

Notice

Knowledge and best practice in this field are constantly changing. As new research and experience
broaden our knowledge, changes in practice, treatment and drug therapy may become necessary or
appropriate. Readers are advised to check the most current information provided (i) on procedures
featured or (ii) by the manufacturer of each product to be administered, to verify the
recommended dose or formula, the method and duration of administration, and contraindications.
It is the responsibility of the practitioner, relying on their own experience and knowledge of the
patient, to make diagnoses, to determine dosages and the best treatment for each individual
patient, and to take all appropriate safety precautions. To the fullest extent of the law, neither the
Publisher nor the Author assumes any liability for any injury and/or damage to persons or property
arising out of or related to any use of the material contained in this book.

The Publisher

Adapted from Crash Course: Imaging, by Barry Kelly and Ian C. Bickle, ISBN: 978-0-7234-3192-3, © 2007.
The rights of Barry Kelly and Ian C. Bickle to be identified as the authors of this book have asserted in
accordance with the Copyright, Designs and Patents Act, 1988.

Library of Congress Cataloging-in-Publication Data

Ter Meulen, Deborah.
  Imaging / Deborah Ter Meulen. -- 1st ed.
    p. ; cm. -- (Crash course)
  Adapted from: Imaging / Barry Kelly, Ian C. Bickle. 2007.
  Includes index.
  ISBN 978-0-323-05338-9
  1. Diagnostic imaging- -Outlines, syllabi, etc. I. Kelly, Barry E. Imaging. II. Title.
III. Series.
  [DNLM: 1. Diagnostic Imaging. WN 180 T315i 2008]
RC78.7.D53T47 2008
  616.07'54- -dc22
                      2007041985

Commissioning Editor: Kate Dimock
Developmental Editor: Andrea Vosburgh
Senior Project Manager: David Saltzberg
Design: Andy Chapman
Cover Design: Antbits Illustration
Illustration Manager: Mick Ruddy

Printed in United States of America

Last digit is the print number: 9 8 7 6 5 4 3 2 1

Preface

Advances in technology have had a huge impact on the practice of medicine. While these advances have impacted many specialties, medical imaging and radiology have benefited the most. Radiology is now critical in the care and management of patients, both diagnostically and therapeutically. Imaging is now commonplace in the evaluation of patients, contemplating physical exams. Similarly, radiology-guided percutaneous treatments (biopsies, drainages, stents, etc.) have replaced many traditional more invasive surgical procedures. This has allowed for more rapid patient convalescence and hence shorter hospital stays. Many procedures can now be done as outpatients.

Radiology has become such an important part of patient care that more medical school programs now include radiology as one of the required clinical rotations. The radiology residency program is also one of the most competitive programs for students to gain acceptance into.

This book aims to provide the basis for diagnostic medical imaging based on organ systems and clinical scenarios most commonly encountered. Within each section, the various imaging tools will be discussed as they pertain to those clinical questions. While some of the therapeutic uses of radiology will be mentioned, the focus of this book is on diagnosis. The concise format of this series will greatly benefit students on their clinical rotations.

Deborah ter Meulen, MD

Dedication

For my family

Contents

Preface v

Part I: The Patient Presents with

1. **Chest Pain, Dyspnea, or Hemoptysis 3**
   Cardiovascular disorders 3
   Respiratory disorders 4
   Case conferences 9

2. **Breast Mass or Breast Screening 13**
   The breast lump 13
   Breast screening 13
   Case conference 14

3. **Dysphagia 15**
   Thyroid mass 15
   Esophageal diseases 15
   Case conference 16

4. **Abdominal Pain 19**
   Imaging in abdominal pain 19
   Intestinal causes 19
   Hepatopancreatobiliary diseases 21
   Urological diseases 22
   Vascular diseases 23
   Gynecological diseases 24
   Case conferences 25

5. **Jaundice 27**
   Liver diseases 27
   Biliary diseases 28
   Pancreatic diseases 29
   Case conference 29

6. **Altered Bowel Habit/Rectal Bleeding 31**
   Small bowel diseases 31
   Large bowel diseases 32
   Case conferences 34

7. **Scrotal or Groin Mass 37**
   Scrotal mass 37
   Inguinal/thigh mass 38
   Case conference 39

8. **Back Pain 41**
   Degenerative diseases 41
   Inflammatory diseases 41
   Neoplastic spinal disease 41

Metabolic bone disease 42
Case conference 44

9. **Joint Pain 47**
   Rheumatoid arthritis 47
   Seronegative arthritis 47
   Degenerative arthritis 48
   Hemophilia 49
   Metabolic disorders 49
   Infectious diseases 50
   Systemic diseases 50
   Case conference 50

10. **Neck Mass 53**
    Thyroid masses 53
    Salivary diseases 54
    Lymphadenopathy 54
    Congenital/developmental diseases 54
    Miscellaneous disorders 55
    Case conference 55

11. **Neurological Symptoms 57**
    Headache 57
    Focal neurological deficit 57
    Seizures 58
    Head trauma 59
    Case conference 61

12. **Urinary Tract Infection in Childhood 63**
    Renal tract ultrasound 63
    Voiding cystourethrogram (VCUG) 63
    DMSA Nuclear study 63
    Other renal imaging investigations used in
    children with UTIs 63
    The role of vesico-ureteric reflux 64
    Case conference 64

13. **Delayed Passage of Meconium 67**
    Hirschsprung's disease 67
    Meconium ileus 67
    Functional immaturity of the colon 67
    Ileal atresia 67
    Anorectal malformations 68
    Colonic atresia 68
    Radiological investigations 68
    Case conference 70

Contents

14. **A Limp in Childhood** **71**
Developmental dysplasia of the hip (DDH) . 71
Transient synovitis of the hip 71
Septic arthritis 71
Perthes' disease 72
Slipped capital femoral epiphysis (SCFE) . . . 72
Toddler's fracture 73
Discitis 73
Radiological evaluation 73
Case conference 74

15. **Pregnancy** **77**
First trimester ultrasound 77
Second trimester ultrasound 78
Third trimester ultrasound 81
Case conference 83

Part II: Principles of Radiology

16. **Ionizing Radiation Studies** **87**
Conventional radiology 87
Computed tomography 90
Interventional radiology 90

17. **Non-ionizing Radiation Techniques** **91**
Ultrasound 91
Doppler ultrasound 91

Magnetic resonance imaging 92

18. **Nuclear Medicine** **93**
Isotopes 93
Single photon emission computed
tomography (SPECT) 93
Positron emission tomography (PET) 93
Specific isotope studies 94
Radiation doses and requests 97

Part III: Image Gallery

19. **Respiratory Imaging** **103**

20. **Cardiovascular and Breast Imaging** **113**

21. **Gastrointestinal Imaging** **121**

22. **Abdominal Imaging** **131**

23. **Orthopedic Imaging** **139**

24. **Head and Neck Imaging** **151**

25. **Pediatric Radiology** **163**

Glossary **173**

Index **175**

THE PATIENT PRESENTS WITH

1. Chest Pain, Dyspnea, or Hemoptysis 3

2. Breast Mass or Breast Screening 13

3. Dysphagia 15

4. Abdominal Pain 19

5. Jaundice 27

6. Altered Bowel Habit/Rectal Bleeding 31

7. Scrotal or Groin Mass 37

8. Back Pain 41

9. Joint Pain 47

10. Neck Mass 53

11. Neurological Symptoms 57

12. Urinary Tract Infection in Childhood 63

13. Delayed Passage of Meconium 67

14. A Limp in Childhood 71

15. Pregnancy 77

1. Chest Pain, Dyspnea, or Hemoptysis

Chest pain, dyspnea, and hemoptysis are frequent reasons for medical admission. With the large prevalence of ischemic heart disease in the western world, acute coronary syndromes should always be at the forefront of the clinician's mind. As the vast majority of chest pain arises from either cardiovascular or respiratory pathology, the plain chest radiograph (CXR) is the usual first-line imaging step.

 Hemoptysis in a smoker over 50 years of age is caused by bronchogenic carcinoma until proven otherwise.

The finding of a normal CXR does not exclude significant pathology. This is particularly the case with pulmonary embolic (PE) disease, the chest radiograph often being unremarkable. Here, the focus moves to appropriate further imaging—either to look for disease not identified on CXR, but for which there is a high clinical suspicion, or to further evaluate an equivocal area of abnormality on plain film. Clearly, particular attention should be paid to excluding an acute cause that would warrant urgent attention, e.g., pneumothorax, dissecting aneurysm, or pericardial tamponade.

 Request an expiratory film if a pneumothorax is suspected. In expiration there is relatively increased intrapleural pressure and the lung edge is maximally displaced from the chest wall.

In many instances, CT of the chest would be the next imaging step—the widened mediastinum on a trauma patient's CXR suggesting aortic dissection; the cavitating mass in the right middle lobe, a bronchogenic carcinoma.

 Squamous cell carcinoma is the most common bronchogenic carcinoma to cavitate.

A VQ scan is more appropriate if the clinical suspicion is of a PE and the CXR is normal. CT pulmonary angiography should be performed if the CXR is abnormal. Although infrequently undertaken by the radiologist, remember the important role of echocardiography and coronary angiography in cardiovascular pathologies—a vital tool in imaging cardiac and pericardial disease.

Cardiovascular disorders

Ischemic heart disease
The chest x-ray is usually normal. However, pacemakers and prosthetic valves are frequent findings. Sternotomy wires and graft clips may be identified. It is also possible to see calcification of the aorta or the left ventricle. This latter feature is usually related to a left ventricular aneurysm.

 The diameter of a prosthetic heart valve is inversely proportional to the pressure across it.

Left ventricular failure
(see Fig. 20.5)

Chest x-ray features (Fig. 1.1) include (as disease progresses):
- Cardiomegaly (cardiothoracic ratio >0.5).
- Increased vascularity to the upper zones and decreased vascularity to the bases.
- Discrete vessels seen in the outer third of the lung fields.

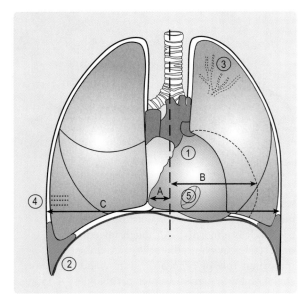

Fig. 1.1 Radiographic features of CHF on CXR: 1. Cardiomegaly (A + B/C = CT ratio > 0.50); 2. Pleural effusion; 3. Upper lobe diversion; 4. Kerley B lines; 5. Possible underlying cause (e.g., mitral valve replacement).

- Kerley B lines at the basal lung periphery (interlobular septal thickening).
- Air space consolidation (pulmonary edema).
- Pleural effusions.

Pericarditis

In acute pericarditis, the chest x-ray is often unremarkable, but radiological signs of pericardial effusion (see Fig. 20.12) would include an enlarged globular or 'water bottle' heart. In the chronic form, pericardial calcification can be seen, especially in the atrioventricular groove and the less pulsatile areas. Sparing of the cardiac apex is a recognized feature.

Aortic dissection

The chest x-ray signs can be conveniently divided into those due to the dissection itself and those due to subsequent rupture.

With dissection, there is:
- Widening of the mediastinum.
- Depression of the left main bronchus.
- Contralateral displacement of a nasogastric (NG) tube (if present).

A useful marker is aortic calcification: if present in the arch on the chest radiograph, this defines the intima. Thus the thickness of the arch wall

(intima–adventitia) can be calculated. Normally this is less than 6 mm. If there is a dissection, it will occur between these layers and therefore the arch wall thickness increases and the calcification is displaced towards the lumen. If the arch wall is of normal thickness, and the NG tube and left main bronchus are normally placed, the possibility of dissection becomes very unlikely.

With rupture, there is evidence of blood in the left chest. This is manifested by apical capping and pleural blood. It is important to remember that if the patient is supine when x-rayed, the pleural blood will lie behind the lung and on the CXR that side will be grayer (less dark) than the other side. This is known as 'veiling' of the lung. In addition, the descending aortic shadow, normally visible behind the heart, will be absent as its silhouette will be obscured (effaced) by blood.

In traumatic transections, the dissection classically occurs at the aortic isthmus—that portion of the aorta just distal to the left subclavian artery where the mobile arch joins the fixed descending thoracic aorta.

On CT scans, the aortic dissection is seen as a flap within the lumen (see Fig. 20.8). Blood is identified around the aorta within the mediastinum (Fig. 1.2). The gold standard investigation is angiography, which will confirm the dissection as a contour abnormality, with contrast accumulation within the dissection or the flap itself; however, multidetector (multislice) CT is increasingly replacing catheter angiography as the definitive diagnostic imaging test.

Respiratory disorders

Pneumonia

Pneumonia typically manifests itself on the CXR as a region of increased density. This density represents the 'consolidated' acini surrounding the air-filled bronchial tree (the 'air bronchogram'). There are four common types of pneumonia in clinical practice: lobar pneumonia, bronchopneumonia, interstitial pneumonia, and cavitating pneumonia.

Lobar pneumonia

Lobar pneumonia affects and therefore delineates a lobe of the lung. The affected lobe can be

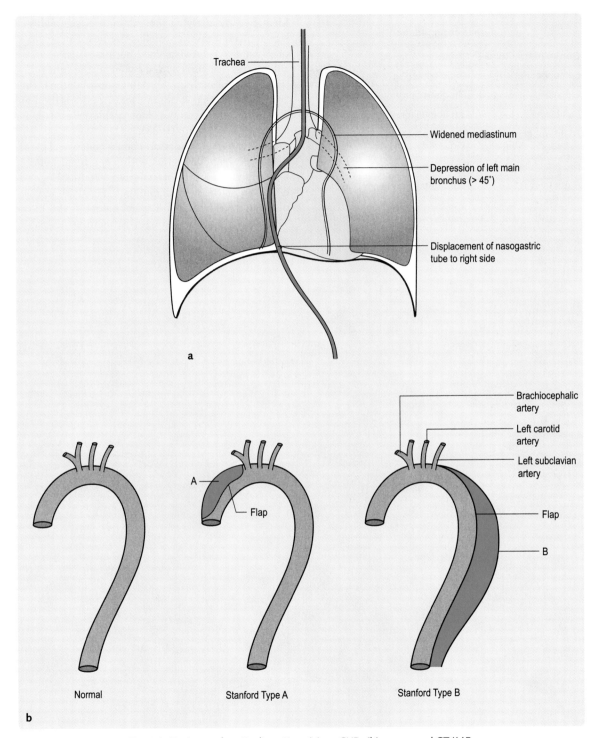

Fig. 1.2 Features of aortic dissection: (a) on CXR; (b) on coronal CT/MR.

Lobar consolidation	
Consolidated lobe	**Structure effaced**
Left upper	Aortic knob (Fig. 1.4a)
Lingula	Left heart border (Fig. 1.4a)
Left lower	Left hemidiaphragm (Fig. 1.4b)
Right upper	Right superior mediastinum (Fig. 1.4e)
Right middle	Right heart border (Fig. 1.4d)
Right lower	Right hemidiaphragm (Fig. 1.4c)

Fig. 1.3 Lobar consolidation.

identified by applying the 'silhouette' sign. This sign indicates that, normally, the heart and diaphragm can be visualized because their silhouettes are surrounded by air in the lungs. If a lobe loses its air (e.g., by being consolidated), then the structure that it abuts cannot be identified and is said to be effaced, i.e., not visible (Figs. 1.3, 1.4; see also Figs. 19.11, 19.23).

Following consolidation comes collapse. This is diagnosed by volume loss within the lung. Left lower lobe collapse, for example, produces elevation of the hemidiaphragm (Fig. 1.5) and depression (downward displacement) of the hilum. The most common pathogen is pneumococcus.

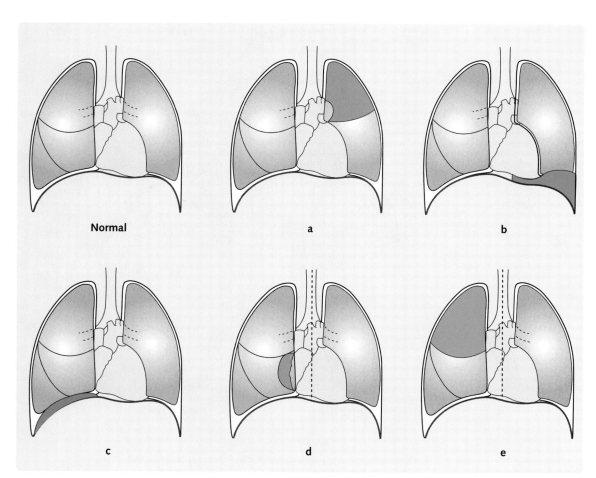

Fig. 1.4 Silhouette signs of consolidation on CXR: (a) left upper lobe (no distinct aortic knob); (b) left lower lobe (loss of left hemidiaphragm silhouette); (c) right lower lobe (loss of right hemidiaphragm); (d) right middle lobe (loss of right heart border); (e) right upper lobe (consolidation limited by horizontal fissure).

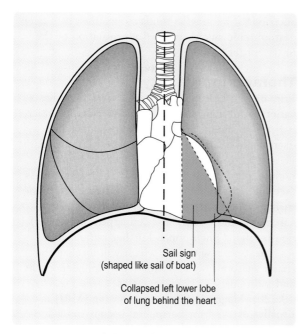

Sail sign
(shaped like sail of boat)

Collapsed left lower lobe
of lung behind the heart

Fig. 1.5 Left lower lobe collapse ('sail' sign).

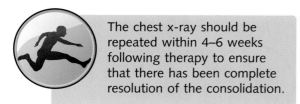

The chest x-ray should be repeated within 4–6 weeks following therapy to ensure that there has been complete resolution of the consolidation.

Bronchopneumonia

The characteristic pattern in bronchopneumonia is multifocal lobular areas of consolidation. These densities are frequently ill defined. 'Spared' or normal lobules between affected areas lead to what has been termed a 'patchwork quilt.' The primary sites of involvement are the terminal and respiratory bronchioles, with disease spreading through the tracheobronchial tree.

Interstitial pneumonia

Interstitial pneumonia usually starts in the bronchus and bronchioles and extends into the interstitium. Interstitial lung disease typically produces widening of the interstitium throughout the lung. These widened structures appear as lines or, when viewed end on, as dots. Therefore, in interstitial pneumonias look for lines and dots throughout the lung. Common causes of interstitial pneumonia are

mycoplasma, chlamydia, and viruses, especially influenza, varicella, and cytomegalovirus. The two most common viral pathogens—varicella and influenza—can present with multifocal consolidation. In the latter case, the consolidation is classically perihilar. Immunosuppressed patients, including those with AIDS, are more susceptible (see Fig. 19.12).

Cavitating pneumonia

Cavitation is seen with many pathogens and can be very difficult to distinguish radiologically from carcinoma. Organisms responsible include staphylococcus, tuberculosis, and klebsiella. Aspiration and Gram-negative pneumonias can also cause cavitation (see Fig. 19.14).

Pulmonary embolus

The chest x-ray is unreliable in the diagnosis of pulmonary embolus (PE) and its main function is to exclude other causes of the patient's symptomatology. However, there are recognized signs of PE on the chest x-ray, the most common being unilateral hypoperfusion (oligemia) in one lung. This is called the Westermark sign.

Ventilation perfusion (VQ) imaging demonstrates an embolism by displaying a region which is ventilated (by the open bronchus) but not perfused (as the artery is occluded by thrombus/embolus). This ventilation–perfusion combination is known as a mismatch. VQ scans are reported as low, intermediate or high probability for PE. The latter two categories usually require treatment. The accuracy of the examination can be undermined by coexistent acute or chronic pulmonary disease. A recent chest radiograph should accompany the patient attending for VQ imaging.

CT scanning

On CT, the embolic material is seen as a black filling defect within the opacified white pulmonary artery (see Fig. 19.20). This is known as the 'polo-mint' sign, seen on axial section. The excellent image resolution of multidetector (multislice) CTs has allowed the diagnosis of pulmonary emboli to be made in smaller segmental arterial branches (Fig. 1.6).

Pneumothorax

The appearances of pneumothorax differ in the erect and the supine chest x-ray (Fig. 1.7). On the

7

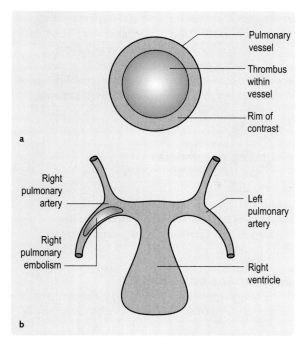

Fig. 1.6 Pulmonary embolus CT: (a) axial with 'polo-mint' sign; (b) longitudinal.

erect film, the pneumothorax is seen as a stripe of air between the lung edge and the chest wall (see Fig. 19.13). It is more clearly appreciated on the expiratory film, as the relatively increased intrapleural pressure maximizes the size of the pneumothorax. On a supine film, the free gas lies anterior to the lung so tends to manifest as a deep costophrenic sulcus or as an accentuation of the heart border.

Thoracic malignancy

Primary thoracic malignancy on chest x-ray has a variety of radiological appearances, none of which is specific, but all are generally suspicious; for example, a hilar mass (see Fig. 19.17), particularly if irregular or spiculated; a solitary pulmonary nodule, particularly if cavitated; or an apical mass (see Fig. 19.16) should all arouse suspicion. Some malignancies, particularly bronchoalveolar carcinoma and lymphoma, can appear as areas of non-resolving pneumonia. Further radiological investigation is with CT, which will localize the lesion anatomically and identify lymphadenopathy and pulmonary or bony metastases (see Fig. 19.22b). Magnetic resonance imaging (MRI) is usually reserved for peripheral lesions to exclude chest wall involvement. Positron emission tomography (PET) scanning is proving effective in confirming the nature of the tumor, staging the disease and identifying recurrent disease in glucose-avid lesions (see Part II, Principles of Radiology).

A calcified lung mass is typically benign.

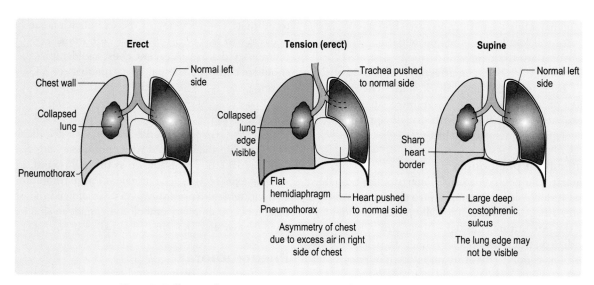

Fig. 1.7 Difference between erect/supine CXR features of pneumothorax.

Metastases

Almost all primary malignancies can metastasize to the lung (see Fig. 19.22a).

Pulmonary metastases are usually seen as multiple circular densities. Common malignancies that metastasize to lung include testicular, renal, thyroid, breast, and colon cancer, lymphomas and sarcomas. Some have relatively specific appearances, e.g., thyroid, which can be tiny and multiple ('miliary') metastases, and renal or sarcomatous metastases ('cannonball'). Calcification is associated with osteogenic sarcoma and colloid metastases, e.g., colon.

Case conferences

Case 1

A 75-year-old male patient is admitted with sudden onset chest pain radiating to the back between the shoulder blades. On examination he is hypertensive (195/99) and a 20 mmHg systolic disparity is noted between the right and left arms. His old medical notes outline a 12-year history of hypertension requiring multiple antihypertensive medications.

Chest x-ray

The heart is enlarged. Pulmonary vascularity is normal, but the mediastinum is widened. The descending aortic shadow is absent. There is no active lung lesion. There is no evidence of an apical cap, nor of a pleural effusion.

CT chest and abdomen

A dynamically enhanced helical CT scan has been performed with contrast administered via the left arm (see Fig. 20.8).

There is an abnormality of the aortic arch with a 'flap' seen beginning distal to the left subclavian artery and extending down the descending thoracic aorta to the upper abdomen. Two lumena—the 'true' and the 'false'—are seen and both are opacified with contrast. There is no abnormality seen relating to the pericardium or ascending arch. There is no pleural fluid collection.

Within the abdomen, contrast opacifies both the celiac and superior mesenteric arteries. Both renal arteries and kidneys are also opacified and, at the level of the renal arteries, the aortic lumen is normal.

Conclusion

The CT appearances are consistent with a Stanford type B aortic dissection. In view of the dissection type, i.e., Stanford type B, the decision is made to manage him conservatively. At outpatient follow-up 3 months later, he is well and normotensive. A follow-up CT scan confirms that the false lumen has occluded.

Case 2

A 70-year-old lady was admitted to the medical ward with an exacerbation of her chronic obstructive pulmonary disease (COPD). Her case was discussed at the weekly radiology meeting. Her initial presentation was with pyrexia, a productive cough and slightly increased dyspnea. The pyrexia and cough had settled with antibiotic therapy but her dyspnea had continued to worsen, despite bronchodilators, physiotherapy, and a trial of steroids.

Initial chest radiograph (on admission)

The heart size and pulmonary vascularity are normal. The lungs are overinflated. Eight anterior ribs are visible in the mid-clavicular line and the hemidiaphragms appear flattened in keeping with the diagnosis of COPD. There was loss of the right hemidiaphragmatic silhouette and an associated area of increased density at the right base. Appearances are consistent with right lower lobe consolidation.

Chest radiograph 3 days later
The appearances are unchanged.

Chest radiograph 2 days later
The right diaphragmatic silhouette remains obscured by the right basal density. In addition there is a meniscus noted peripherally, extending up along the lateral chest wall to the apex. This latter appearance is consistent with a pleural effusion.

The physician then informs the meeting that the clinical appearances were also consistent with a right-sided pleural effusion. He consults the radiologist for advice regarding further imaging and intervention.

Ultrasound chest
A large anechoic (dark) area is noted above the diaphragm with a central echogenic triangular zone. There were no septations visible. The ultrasonic image is consistent with a large pleural effusion. The central zone represents consolidated lung.

Because of the clinical concern regarding underlying malignancy, in consultation with the radiologists, the decision was made to undergo CT of the chest, with a view to possible CT guided drainage.

CT chest
The initial set of images confirm the right lower lobe consolidation, with an associated low attenuation zone peripherally, consistent with the known pleural effusion. No mass lesion or endobronchial stenosis is seen.
The second set demonstrates the patient has been turned into the prone position.

A needle is identified, the tip of which lies in the pleural collection. Subsequent images show that a wire and finally a 12F pigtail catheter are located within the collection.

The physician informs you that the procedure was routine, and that straw-colored aspirate was drained. Biochemical and microbiological analysis revealed a sterile exudative pleural effusion. The patient's dyspnea improved dramatically overnight, and the fluid was sent for cytological evaluation.*

Case 3
A 24-year-old male patient was transferred from the orthopedic unit to the medical admissions unit 2 days ago following an episode of hemoptysis.

He had been admitted to hospital 10 days earlier following a fractured right femur sustained when his bicycle had been involved in a road traffic accident with a car. His right femur had been treated by open reduction and internal fixation with an intramedullary nail.

On examination he was dyspneic with a tachycardia of 120 bpm. His blood pressure is 103/50. ECG reveals right bundle branch block and a sinus tachycardia. An arterial blood gas sample confirms a type 1 respiratory failure picture with a PaO_2 of 7.9 kPa on 50% oxygen. There is no evidence of an axillary rash.

Chest x-ray
Heart size and pulmonary vascularity are normal. No active lung lesion. Normal chest radiograph.

VQ scan
There is an area of mismatch at the right lung base. Appearances are suspicious of a pulmonary embolus (intermediate/high probability). CT recommended to confirm the diagnosis of pulmonary embolus.

*Cytological evaluation showed no evidence of malignancy. The effusion was para-pneumonic in nature. The patient made an excellent recovery and was discharged.

CT scan

A dynamically enhanced multidetector CT scan was performed using the pulmonary angiographic algorithm. The pulmonary conus and main pulmonary arteries enhance normally. A central filling defect is noted in the right descending pulmonary artery. The appearance of this defect—the 'polo-mint' sign—is consistent with a pulmonary embolus in the right descending pulmonary artery.

He is commenced on therapeutic low molecular weight heparin (LMWH) and warfarinized. When the INR was greater than 2.0, his LMWH was discontinued and he was discharged on warfarin with suitable follow-up arrangements in place.

2. Breast Mass or Breast Screening

Focal breast lesions may present in three ways: the mass may be discovered by the patient on breast self-examination (BSE), by a doctor during a clinical breast examination (CBE), or as part of a breast screening program. Breast screening programs begin with mammography, but may proceed to assessment with additional view mammography, ultrasound, or breast MRI (Fig. 2.1). Furthermore, imaging may also be used to guide biopsy either by ultrasound, stereotaxis, or MRI.

The breast lump

Management of the symptomatic breast lump depends on the patient's age.

The patient is under 35 years of age
Following clinical examination, the first imaging modality used is ultrasound. If the lesion is cystic, then typically no further intervention is necessary. If the lesion is solid, fine needle aspiration (FNA) or core biopsy is performed. The most common solid mass in this age group is a benign fibroadenoma (see Fig. 20.16).

The patient is 35 years of age or older
The preliminary imaging technique is mammography (using craniocaudal and lateral oblique projections). If a focal mass is identified on the mammogram, then ultrasound of the lesion follows. If the lesion proves cystic, then aspiration is performed. If the lesion is solid on ultrasound (see Fig. 20.17), then FNA is performed. Should mammography identify microcalcification (see Fig. 20.21), then a stereotactic core biopsy of the area is performed to exclude breast carcinoma.

Breast screening

The National Cancer Institute (NCI) recommends screening for breast cancer with breast self examination (BSE), clinical breast examination (CBE) by a physician, and yearly mammograms.

The screening mammogram consists of two views of each breast (mediolateral oblique [MLO] and craniocaudal [CC]). The mammogram is interpreted by a radiologist. In most cases, the examination will be normal and the patient will be asked to return for a mammogram in one year. If there is an abnormality on the screening study (see Figs. 20.18 to 20.21), the patient will be called back for additional imaging. At this time the radiologist will supervise additional mammographic imaging (magnification or spot compression views), perform an ultrasound, and/or recommend an MRI of the breasts.

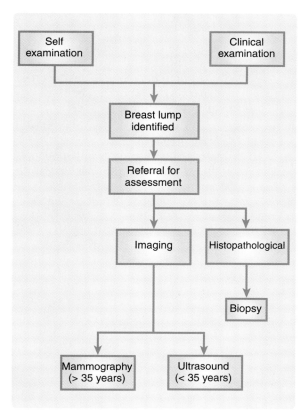

Fig. 2.1 Algorithm for breast lump assessment.

If the abnormality persists, e.g., evidence of a solid mass (see Figs. 20.16, 20.18), parenchymal distortion (see Figs. 20.19, 20.22), or abnormal patterns of calcification (see Fig. 20.21), an image guided FNA or core biopsy can be performed. This can be done under ultrasound, MRI, or stereotactic guidance. MR guided biopsies are usually only performed if the lesion cannot be seen by ultrasound or mammography, only on MRI.

Depending on the pathology results, there are three possibilities: surgery, short term follow-up (usually 6 months), or routine yearly follow-up.

Breast carcinoma is the second most common malignancy in women in the US.

Case conference

A 54-year-old lady was referred by her general practitioner with a mass in the upper outer quadrant of her left breast. Her menopause was at the age of 51 years. She has noticed the lump over the past 4 weeks while showering. On examination, a firm, 2 cm, fixed mass was noted in the upper outer quadrant. The contralateral breast and the axillae were unremarkable. Examination of the cervical lymph nodes, abdomen, and spine was normal.

Mammogram
Craniocaudal and mediolateral images of the left breast were reviewed. In the upper outer quadrant of the left breast, there is a spiculated lesion with microcalcification.

No other lesion is seen. The appearances are very suspicious of a carcinoma, and ultrasound guided FNA is recommended.

Ultrasound
Under ultrasound guidance, the lesion in the left breast was identified, confirmed to be solid, and biopsied. The cytologist confirmed the radiologist's diagnosis of carcinoma.

Conclusion
Her case was discussed at the weekly multidisciplinary meeting and surgery was scheduled for the following week. A wide local excision with axillary node dissection was undertaken. Adjuvant chemotherapy in the form of anastrozole was commenced.

3. Dysphagia

In dysphagia, clinical examination is of limited value, and generally medical imaging or endoscopy is required to make a definitive diagnosis.

Plain chest radiographs are occasionally able to identify pathology, such as achalasia or a hiatus hernia. The mainstay of imaging is with upper gastrointestinal contrast studies, usually with barium, although on occasion with a water-soluble agent if perforation is suspected (barium causes a severe mediastinitis if it leaks). CT is generally reserved for tumor staging or surveillance. In the case of esophageal carcinoma, endoluminal ultrasound is a developing area in the assessment of tumor depth, and thus potential for surgery.

PET has a growing role in the staging of esophageal malignancy.

A retrosternal thyroid mass is a differential diagnosis for an anterior mediastinal mass on CXR.

Achalasia is a predisposing factor for esophageal carcinoma.

There are two main causes of dysphagia: thyroid masses and esophageal diseases.

Thyroid mass

The chest x-ray (CXR) may show contralateral displacement of the trachea by a thyroid mass (benign or malignant). X-rays of the thoracic inlet (AP and lateral views) will show tracheal displacement and narrowing.

Ultrasound demonstrates enlargement of the thyroid, the size and consistency of focal thyroid masses, and any associated lymphadenopathy.

Isotope thyroid studies will identify 'hot' and 'cold' lesions. 'Cold' lesions have an association with malignancy: for a single nodule, 15–25%; for multiple nodules 1–6%. CT assesses retrosternal extension and, if carcinoma is suspected, lymphadenopathy and metastatic tumor spread.

Metastatic pulmonary lesions from thyroid carcinoma produce a 'miliary' appearance on chest x-ray (as may histoplasmosis and TB).

Esophageal diseases

Esophageal web
Barium swallow demonstrates a fine anterior transverse filling defect in the upper esophageal lumen (see Fig. 21.4). Clinical associations of webs include Plummer–Vinson (Paterson–Brown Kelly) syndrome.

Pharyngeal pouch
Barium swallow shows a pouch containing barium and food debris at the upper end of the esophagus (see Fig. 21.8). The pouch is found at Killian's dehiscence, which is between the thyropharyngeus and cricopharyngeus fibers of the inferior constrictor muscle (see also Ch. 10).

Esophageal candidiasis
Barium swallow reveals an irregular mucosa with multiple filling defects (see Fig. 21.3). This is more commonly diagnosed at endoscopy.

Achalasia
CXR demonstrates a dilated esophagus, often with a fluid level. The gastric air bubble is classically absent. There may also be evidence of repeated

pulmonary aspiration with fibrotic changes in the dependent lung.

Barium reveals a dilated esophagus with a smoothly tapering lower end. Irregular stricturing suggests malignant transformation (see Figs 21.1, 21.2).

Hiatus hernia
Chest x-ray demonstrates a retrocardiac air-filled structure, on occasion with a fluid level (see Fig. 21.12). A left lateral film will confirm its location and the diagnosis.

Barium swallow will show the location and the extent of the hernia, and confirm the presence of gastro-esophageal reflux disease (GERD).

Hiatus hernias can be subdivided into sliding (80%) and rolling or paraesophageal hernias (20%).

Esophageal varices
Although endoscopy is now the primary imaging modality, barium studies reveal serpiginous filling defects along the long axis of the esophagus, particularly in the prone position (see Fig. 21.6). Ultrasound will show the hepatic architecture, particularly cirrhosis, focal liver lesions, splenomegaly, and ascites. CT will confirm the ultrasound findings, as well as aberrant vessels (e.g., splanchnic varices, portal venous transformation, the periumbilical 'caput medusae') and focal liver lesions (e.g., hepatoma).

Look for associated clinical signs of chronic liver disease, chiefly splenomegaly.

Esophageal corrosive stricture
This follows ingestion of corrosive liquids. Barium studies show a long smooth tapering stricture (see Fig. 21.5).

A long, gently tapered stricture is nearly always benign.

Esophageal carcinoma
CXR is insensitive at diagnosing an esophageal carcinoma unless the proximal esophagus is distended, in which case a fluid level may be appreciable. However, pulmonary and skeletal metastases may be appreciated, as may evidence of previous surgery, e.g., total esophagectomy, in which case there is a widened mediastinum due to the transposed stomach and an absent gastric air bubble in the left hypochondrium.

Barium swallow shows an irregular shouldered stricture—'the rat's tail' (see Fig. 21.7). An associated hiatus hernia suggests that the carcinoma may have resulted from area of Barrett's esophagus secondary to reflux. This would be an adenocarcinoma. CT is used to stage the disease and identify nodes, tumor fixity and metastatic spread. PET scanning is gaining increased acceptance as the staging test for esophageal disease. Endoluminal ultrasound is helpful in assessing the depth of tumor invasion.

A history of chronic reflux with Barrett's esophagus is significant in the development of adenocarcinoma of the lower third of the esophagus.

Case conference

A 68-year-old lady presented to the gastroenterologists with a 3-month history of increasingly progressive dysphagia. She had lost 10 kg in weight. She has an extensive smoking history. On examination, she was cachexic. No fasciculations were seen and cranial nerves were intact.

CXR

Cardiac contour and pulmonary vascularity are normal. There is an area of scarring at the right apex. No other pulmonary abnormality is seen.

Barium swallow

There is a 4 cm long strictured area with loss of the normal esophageal mucosa. 'Shouldering' is noted at the edges of the stricture. Barium passes beyond the stricture into the distal esophagus and stomach. The stomach and duodenum outline normally. The appearances are consistent with an esophageal carcinoma.

CT scan

A dynamically enhanced multidetector CT scan was performed through the chest and upper abdomen. There is dilatation of the upper esophagus with an abrupt change in caliber at the level of the carina, corresponding to an endoscopic level of 28 cm. Fat planes are preserved around the esophagus. There are two nodes present in the mediastinum, both less than 1 cm in diameter. An area of fibrotic parenchymal scarring is identified in the right upper lobe bronchus. There was no definite pulmonary mass lesion.

Within the abdomen the liver, adrenal glands, pancreas, spleen, and kidneys are normal. There is no significant adenopathy or ascites.

Conclusion

The appearances are consistent with an esophageal mass lesion. Two mediastinal lymph nodes are identified, as is an area of fibrosis in the right upper lobe. The abdomen is normal. PET–CT is recommended for further staging.

PET–CT scan

A whole body PET–CT scan was performed following the IV administration of [18]FDG. A glucose-avid lesion is identified in the esophagus at the level of the carina. There is no isotope uptake in the mediastinum or right apex. No other glucose-avid lesion is demonstrated.

The appearances are consistent with an esophageal carcinoma. There is no evidence of disease outside the esophagus.

She is referred back to the gastroenterologists for consideration for surgery.

4. Abdominal Pain

Imaging in abdominal pain

The differential diagnosis for abdominal pain is immense. There are many imaging tests at one's disposal. The judicious use of these will depend on a thorough patient examination, and the clinical impression of the underlying pathology will dictate the imaging direction, e.g., loin pain and hematuria—urological; right upper quadrant pain in an overweight 43-year-old lady—hepatobiliary; central abdominal pain radiating to the back in an arteriopath—aortic aneurysm.

Plain abdominal radiographs are useful for evaluating gas, both intraluminal and extraluminal, and calculi.

Ultrasound is sensitive in the evaluation of any fluid-filled structure, excellent at detecting calculi and good at evaluation of solid organs. A kidney obstructed by calculus with a resultant hydronephrosis is elegantly demonstrated by ultrasound. On the other hand, ultrasound is very insensitive in the evaluation of gaseous structures, as the sound waves are reflected by air. Searching for a duodenal ulcer with ultrasound is a fruitless task!

Computed tomography (CT) has all the advantages of plain radiographs and ultrasound. So, why not use it for everything? The radiation dose generated by CT is large and must be clinically justified.

The likelihood of anyone contracting a malignancy from the Earth's background radiation is 1: 1,000,000. Following a CT of the abdomen, this rises to 1: 2000. Furthermore, the risk rises with successive scans, no matter whether they are performed the next day or 20 years later. On the other hand, the risk of contracting a malignancy during one's life is 1: 3. It all comes down to relative risk. How sick is the patient? How old is the patient? Can the imaging be acquired by alternative methodology, e.g., ultrasound, MRI, or endoscopy?

Systems which cause abdominal pain are:
- Intestinal.
- Hepatopancreatobiliary.
- Urological.
- Vascular.
- Gynecological.
- Miscellaneous.

Intestinal causes

- Large bowel obstruction.
- Small bowel obstruction.
- Volvulus.
- Pseudo-obstruction.
- Diverticulosis.
- Pneumoperitoneum.
- Intestinal ischemia.
- Appendicitis.

Large bowel obstruction

On the abdominal x-ray (AXR) there are dilated large bowel loops, with haustral markings evident, which occupy a peripheral location on the film (see Fig. 21.22). A cut-off point may be apparent, as may small bowel dilatation, if there is an associated incompetent ileocecal valve.

Contrast studies will identify the level of bowel obstruction. Barium is used primarily unless there is a significant risk of perforation, in which case water-soluble contrast, such as hypaque or iopamidol (Niopam), may be substituted. CT will demonstrate change in bowel caliber and the level of obstruction. The underlying etiology such as a colonic mass may be identified (Fig. 4.1). In such cases, lymphadenopathy and metastatic disease can also be excluded.

Polyp size and malignant transformation	
Size (cm)	Risk of malignant transformation
<0.5	Rarely malignant
<1	1%
1–2	10%
>2	50%

Fig. 4.1 Polyp size and malignant transformation.

Comparison of radiological features of small and large bowel obstruction		
Radiological feature	Small bowel obstruction	Large bowel obstruction
Bowel diameter	<5 cm	>5 cm
Location	Central	Peripheral
Haustra	No	Yes
Valvulae	Yes	No
Large bowel gas	No	Yes, look for 'cut-off'

Fig. 4.2 Comparison of radiological features of small and large bowel obstruction.

Small bowel obstruction

The AXR demonstrates dilated small bowel loops and these occupy a central position on the film (see Fig. 21.15). Valvulae conniventes will be evident, confirming the small bowel nature of the loops. The number of loops is dependent on the level of obstruction within small bowel (e.g., few loops in a high, proximal obstruction). Fluid levels are present on the upright AXR (see Fig. 21.16). A small bowel series with dilute barium identifies the level of obstruction, although if complete obstruction is suspected, a water-soluble contrast such as gastrografin or iopamidol may be more appropriate (Fig. 4.2). CT identifies the level of the obstruction and may determine the likely etiology, e.g., Crohn's disease with a stricture and inflammatory changes in the surrounding fatty tissues.

> The most common causes of small bowel obstruction are adhesions, hernias, and lesions *outside* the small bowel—look for abdominal surgery scars and check the hernial orifices. The most common causes of large bowel obstruction are adhesions, lesions *inside* the large bowel, and hernias.

Volvulus

Volvulus occurs when a loop of gastrointestinal tract twists about its mesentery. The most common sites are at the stomach, the cecum and the sigmoid colon. Gastric volvulus is described according to the axis of the 'twist' and is classified as organoaxial or mesenteroaxial. Presentation is with epigastric or chest pain.

Cecal volvulus obstructs the terminal ileum, so presents as a small bowel obstruction (see Fig. 21.15). The cecum often lies in the left or right upper quadrant and is absent from its normal location ('empty cecum' sign). Sigmoid volvulus, which characteristically occurs in the more elderly population, presents as a large bowel obstruction (see Fig. 21.23). The twisted loops of the sigmoid colon converge about its mesentery ('coffee-bean' sign). Contrast enema will confirm the sigmoid obstruction, and has a characteristic beak appearance.

Pseudo-obstruction

AXR identifies small and large bowel dilatation, with no cut-off point. This often follows surgery. A contrast study of the colon will confirm the lack of a 'cut-off' point.

Diverticulosis

The AXR is usually normal. There may be evidence of the complications of diverticular disease, e.g., large bowel obstruction or perforation. The radiological investigation of choice is a contrast enema. Contrast collects in bowel outpouchings (diverticula) (see Fig. 21.17). Evidence of complications, such as stricture and perforation, are also detectable. CT not only confirms the enema findings, but also allows the anatomical delineation of complications (fistulae, strictures, abscess) and image-guided drainage of collections.

> Diverticula protrude *outside* the bowel wall and can fill with contrast. Polyps protrude *inside* the bowel lumen and cause a filling defect within the contrast.

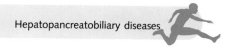

Pneumoperitoneum

On the upright chest or abdominal radiograph, free gas is seen beneath the hemidiaphragm(s). On a supine abdominal projection, various radiological signs have been described. These include the falciform ligament sign and Rigler's sign (see Figs 21.9–21.11).

A water-soluble contrast study may detect the leakage of contrast through the perforated bowel wall; however, with a duodenal ulcer, the perforation may quickly be sealed by omentum. A negative study therefore does not exclude the diagnosis. Endoscopy is the investigation of choice. US will identify free fluid, especially in the subhepatic and pelvic areas. A CT scan will confirm an extravisceral collection, especially useful if the perforation has sealed.

The most common viscera to perforate are the duodenum (ulcer) and the sigmoid colon (diverticulum).

Be aware of Chilaiditi's sign—gas beneath the diaphragm which on close inspection has haustral markings and represents normal intraluminal bowel air, not a perforation.

Causes of pneumoperitoneum: perforated viscus, post-laparotomy/oscopy.

Intestinal ischemia

The AXR demonstrates bowel distension and 'thumbprinting' (see Fig. 21.24). However, 'thumbprinting' is not a specific sign of bowel ischemia. The splenic flexure is the most common site in ischemic colitis. With disease progression, mural and portal venous gas may be appreciated on plain radiographs, the latter sign being very ominous. CT will confirm these features. Other associated pathology may be identified, such as vascular calcification, thrombosis, ascites, and visceral perforation.

Appendicitis

On the AXR an appendicolith is seen as a radio-opacity in the right lower quadrant. This finding is present in 14% of cases. US can be used to measure the appendiceal diameter (normal < 6 mm) and occasionally to view an appendicolith. This is of particular value in children and young adults. Although CT is not often clinically indicated in these patients, an appendicolith is seen as an intraluminal appendicular calcified mass. Appendicular thickening, inflammation of the surrounding fat planes and free intraperitoneal fluid can also be appreciated.

Appendicitis is essentially a clinical diagnosis.

Contrast studies are contraindicated in intestinal ischemia due to the risk of bowel perforation.

Hepatopancreatobiliary diseases

- Cholelithiasis.
- Acute pancreatitis.
- Chronic pancreatitis.
- Biliary colic.

Cholelithiasis and biliary colic

Calcified gallstones are seen in the right upper quadrant on AXR in 10–20% of cases as laminated structures of varying size (see Fig. 22.10). US is the investigation of choice, with gallstones seen as bright (echogenic) structures with an associated dark posterior band (the acoustic shadow, Fig. 4.3). Any biliary dilatation will also be evident. The diameter of the common hepatic duct at the porta hepatis is typically ≤ 6 mm. However it is known to enlarge by 1 mm per decade after 40 years of age, and also is larger in patients with a previous history of cholecystectomy.

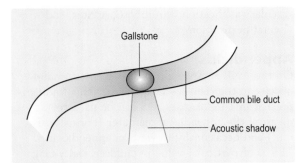

Fig. 4.3 Ultrasound of a stone in the bile duct, showing the acoustic shadow effect.

CT may demonstrate the calculus (if its attenuation value is higher than bile) and any significant biliary dilatation. Other complications of obstructing biliary calculus, e.g. pancreatitis with glandular enlargement, surrounding inflammatory changes and ascites, will be identified.

On MRI, gallstones appear as low signal within the high signal gallbladder bile on T2 weighted (T2W) sequences. Magnetic resonance cholangiography (MRC) superbly visualizes duct caliber and has the advantage of no associated radiation (see Fig. 22.21). ERCP should now be reserved for interventional cases, such as sphincterotomy, stone removal and stent placement (see Fig. 22.9).

Acute pancreatitis

On AXR a sentinel loop and 'cut-off' sign are classically seen. The underlying cause may be apparent, e.g., gallstones.

Ultrasound will detect gallstones, as well as any increase in size or irregularity of the pancreas, although the pancreas can be difficult to view due to obscuring bowel gas. Complications of pancreatitis, including pseudocyst and ascites, are detectable. CT will demonstrate an enlarged and/or edematous pancreas. Necrosis and pancreatic pseudocysts are clearly outlined (see Figs 22.4, 22.5).

The US identification of gallstones is frequently coincidental. It may not explain the patient's symptomatology. Clinical correlation is paramount.

CT needs to be performed with IV contrast enhancement to detect pancreatic necrosis.

Chronic pancreatitis

The AXR demonstrates speckled calcification transversely across the upper abdomen in the pancreatic distribution (see Fig. 22.6). CT shows pancreatic calcification, along with atrophy of the gland and a dilated pancreatic duct. MRC demonstrates pancreatic duct morphology.

Urological diseases

- Renal colic.
- Renal malignancy.
- Urinary tract infection.

Renal colic

The incidence of renal calculus is 7 per 1000 of the population, with an overall lifetime risk of 40–60% (male: female ratio 2: 1). Renal calculi are visible on plain abdominal radiographs in up to 60% of cases. Other evidence of the underlying cause, e.g., hyperparathyroidism, may be present, i.e., osteopenic vertebral bodies and vascular calcification. The intravenous pyelogram (IVP) has traditionally been the gold standard in identifying the presence of calculus and level of ureteric obstruction. The obstructed kidney opacifies later than the normal side. There is delayed filling of the pelvicalyceal system and the calyces are swollen and blunted ('clubbed').

Ultrasound scan, as with gallstones, shows the calculus with its posterior acoustic shadowing but is sensitive in only 40–60% of cases. Calyceal dilatation may be seen proximal to the obstructing calculus. Unenhanced CT identifies renal calculus in 99% of cases. Dilatation of the renal tract proximal to the calculus may be evident. CT urography is gaining acceptance as the first-line investigation in renal colic.

Beware of phleboliths on abdominal radiographs. These are small, smooth, circular venous calcifications. Classically they lie below the level of the ischial spines.

Never comment on an IVP without the preliminary scout film.

Renal malignancy

The most common renal malignancy is renal cell carcinoma. Rarely the AXR may show displacement of adjacent structures, e.g., bowel, by the tumor. Evidence of metastatic bony involvement may be seen as lucent, expansile deposits within the bones. However, the AXR appearances are often normal.

US typically reveals a solid renal mass. Tumor extension into the renal vein and inferior vena cava may be delineated, as may liver metastases. CT demonstrates a solid renal mass (see Fig. 22.7b) and any extension into adjacent structures, particularly the renal vein and inferior vena cava. CT is the gold standard for tumor staging.

If renal malignancy is detected, obtain a chest radiograph to exclude cannonball metastases.

If left-sided testicular varicocele is the primary diagnosis, check for renal malignancy on US. The left gonadal vein drains into the left renal vein and can be obstructed by invading left-sided renal tumor.

Urinary tract infection

This is essentially a clinical diagnosis. US is used to look for any underlying cause—calculus, obstruction, evidence of chronicity, scarring or cortical thinning. Nuclear medicine (DMSA) scans are useful for differential renal function and demonstrating renal scarring (see also Ch. 12), and DTPA renograms for excluding renal outlet obstruction.

Vascular diseases

- Abdominal aortic aneurysm.
- Aortic dissection.
- Intestinal ischemia.

Abdominal aortic aneurysm

The AXR may demonstrate an aneurysm as a curvilinear central or paravertebral calcification with loss of parallelism of the aortic walls (Fig. 4.4). Look for calcification of other vessels. US can accurately measure the transverse dimensions of the aneurysm and the relationship to the neck of the renal arteries (supra-, juxta-, and infrarenal). Evidence of para-aortic rupture is detectable.

Contrast enhanced CT is the gold standard for measuring aneurysm dimensions, assessing the relationship with the renal arteries, the nature of the aneurysm (fusiform, saccular) and the caliber of the iliac vessels distal to the aneurysm (Fig. 4.5). It is the gold standard for identifying an aortic leak. Helical and multidetector (multislice) CT imaging

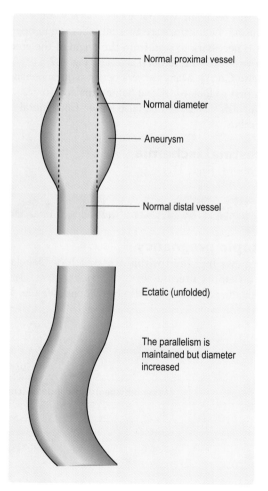

Normal proximal vessel

Normal diameter

Aneurysm

Normal distal vessel

Ectatic (unfolded)

The parallelism is maintained but diameter increased

Fig. 4.4 The difference between an ectatic and an aneurysmal aorta.

Normal aortic diameter	
Vertebral level	Normal aortic diameter (cm)
T12	2.5
L2	2.0
L4	1.5

Fig. 4.5 Normal aortic diameter.

Stanford classification of thoracic aortic dissection		
Type	Origin	Treatment
A	Ascending aortic arch	Surgical
B	Distal to subclavian artery	Conservative

Fig. 4.7 Stanford classification of thoracic aortic dissection.

is important in the planning of aortic stent patients (Fig. 4.6; see also Fig. 20.11).

Aortic dissection
CT delineates the origin and length of the dissection and identifies the true and false aneurysm lumina. It confirms renal and visceral artery patency and perfusion. Dissections are typically thoracic in origin so it is necessary to scan from the origin of the great arch vessels to the femoral arteries (Fig. 4.7; see also Ch. 1). Many centers perform an unenhanced scan first to look for mural hematoma and to distinguish slow flow in a false lumen from mural thrombus.

Intestinal ischemia
See above, page 21.

Gynecological diseases

Ectopic pregnancy
US shows free fluid within the pouch of Douglas and an empty uterus.
An adnexal mass may also be evident (see Ch. 15).

Fibroids (leiomyomata)
The AXR may show a discrete calcified pelvic lesion. US identifies discrete, solid, hypoechoic and sometimes multiple uterine masses. On MRI, simple fibroids are seen as discrete, solid, low signal masses on T1W and T2W sequences. Heterogeneous areas of high signal on the T2W are associated with fibroid degeneration.

Torsion of ovarian cyst
US will demonstrate pelvic free fluid and an adnexal cystic mass.

Endometriosis
US is used first line to detect the solid and cystic mass(es) of endometriosis. These are seen most commonly on the ovary and broad ligament. Chocolate cysts (endometriomas) on MRI have a distinct signal pattern due to the blood breakdown products.

Abdominal/pelvic abscess
Displacement of adjacent structures can be seen on AXR and air fluid levels on erect films. US demonstrates cystic and complex fluid collections

Surveillance of AAA	
Maximum aneurysm diameter (cm)	Action
3.5–4.5	Annual US scan
4.6–5.5	6-monthly US scan review
>5.5	Consider surgery/endovascular repair

Fig. 4.6 Surveillance of AAA.

and is useful for planning guided intervention. CT outlines the same features as US but may also indicate associated pathology or cause, e.g., diverticular disease, pancreatitis.

Pelvic inflammatory disease

This is primarily a clinical diagnosis in women of childbearing age. US is used to exclude complications, e.g., hydrosalpinx and pyosalpinx.

Transvaginal US gives better image resolution of the uterus and ovaries than transabdominal US, but is a more invasive (and intimate) examination.

Case conferences

Case 1

A 56-year-old woman presented last night with abdominal pain and vomiting that she had had for about a week, gradually getting worse. She has a history of surgery for removal of a carcinoid tumor of the terminal ileum 5 years previously. She has been well ever since.

Plain radiographs

Abdominal radiographs demonstrate multiple distended loops of bowel. These are located centrally within the abdomen, and the presence of valvulae conniventes confirms them as small bowel loops. There is no gas in the colon or rectum.

The appearances are consistent with mechanical small bowel obstruction.

Small bowel series

There are distended loops of small bowel. There was no progression of contrast into the large bowel. The appearances are consistent with mechanical small bowel obstruction.

CT abdomen

CT of the abdomen with IV contrast demonstrates an irregular mass lesion in the right iliac fossa invading the adjacent bowel mesentery. Distended loops of small bowel are confirmed. Large bowel diameter is normal. There are multiple low attenuation lesions within both lobes of the liver.

The appearances are consistent with a malignant tumor mass invading the mesentery and causing small bowel obstruction. There are also multiple liver metastases.

Given the known history of terminal ileal carcinoid, the diagnosis could be confirmed by octreotide (sandostatin) nuclear medicine imaging.

Case 2

A 53-year-old lady was referred by her general practitioner with a 7-month history of lower abdominal pain and intermittent vaginal bleeding. She had been climacteric for the past 14 months. History was otherwise unremarkable. No significant abnormality was found on abdominal examination. Per vaginal examination: no mass lesion or discharge noted.

Abdominal radiograph

The bowel gas pattern is unremarkable with no evidence of intestinal obstruction or perforation. There is no evidence of renal or ureteric calculi. A 4 cm circular calcific density is noted centrally within the pelvis.

Ultrasound of abdomen and pelvis

The gallbladder, liver, biliary tree, and pancreas outline normally. Both kidneys are sonographically normal with no evidence of calculus, hydronephrosis, or mass lesion.

Above the bladder, the uterus is prominent and there is a 4 cm mass with posterior acoustic shadowing noted within it. The appearances are consistent with those seen on the abdominal radiograph, and are very suggestive of a calcified fibroid.

MR pelvis

Axial, sagittal, and coronal T2W sequences, along with sagittal T1W and STIR (fat suppression), are available for review. There is a focal mass measuring 4.1 cm in diameter seen within the dorsal uterine wall on all sequences. The characteristics are of a low signal lesion on all pulse sequences, and the appearance is consistent with a uterine fibroid. No other significant abnormality is seen.

This lady's gynecologist informed her of these reassuring findings and management options. She chose medical management with follow-up at outpatients.

5. Jaundice

Jaundice is a presenting symptom crossing medical and surgical specialties, its underlying causes ranging from the entirely reversible (biliary calculi) to the fatal (pancreatic cancer). It is in delineating these pathologies that imaging has a pivotal role—establishing the etiology and thus the correct treatment modality. Increasingly the radiologist has the primary interventional role in the management of hepatobiliary malignancies.

There are several imaging investigations available for the assessment of the jaundiced patient and a logical sequence in which to use them based on clinical and biochemical findings. Ultrasound, CT, MRC, and PTC are all helpful in different ways, supplemented by ERCP, which has both a diagnostic and a therapeutic role. The choice of initial investigation should be guided by clinical acumen. The middle aged, overweight, Caucasian lady with right upper quadrant pain is likely to have gallstone disease, making ultrasound appropriate initially. On the other hand, a 75-year-old man with deep, painless jaundice, 10 kg of weight loss, and an elevated CA 19-9 tumor marker is more likely to require a CT abdomen to exclude pancreatic carcinoma.

Liver diseases

Hepatitis
On ultrasound, acute hepatitis generally has no distinguishing features. Chronic hepatitis has appearances similar to cirrhosis.

Cirrhosis
Radiologically, the appearances reflect two stages in the disease: fatty change and fibrosis. A fatty liver is enlarged or normal in size. On ultrasound, fatty liver is coarse with decreased penetration and, when fibrotic, is shrunken with an irregular margin. CT of the fatty liver shows an enlarged, low attenuation (dark) organ. In advanced disease, the liver becomes small. The margins may be irregular, and sparing of the caudate lobe is characteristic.

In chronic cirrhosis, careful evaluation of the liver must be made for a focal hepatic mass, i.e., a regenerating nodule or, more worryingly, the development of a hepatocellular carcinoma.

The focal liver lesion
There are six commonly occurring liver lesions which, although not necessarily associated with jaundice, constitute a significant proportion of a radiologist's working practice. A detailed description of these is beyond the scope of this book, but some basic principles apply.

The lesions are (see Fig. 22.15):
- Simple hepatic cyst.
- Hemangioma.
- Hepatic adenoma.
- Focal nodular hyperplasia.
- Hepatocellular carcinoma.
- Metastases.

Simple hepatic cyst
This is the most common focal hepatic 'mass' detected. On ultrasound, it is completely dark ('anechoic'), with a bright tail ('through enhancement') deep to it. It is of low attenuation on CT (< 15 Hounsfield units) and does not enhance with IV contrast. On MR a cyst is of low signal on T1W and high signal on T2W sequences. Its signal will be identical to the CSF within the spinal canal.

Hemangioma
A common incidental finding in cross-sectional imaging studies and on ultrasound, a hemangioma is typically brighter (hyperechoic) than the surrounding liver parenchyma. On unenhanced CT, hemangiomas are of lower attenuation (i.e., darker) than the surrounding liver. However, within a few minutes of contrast administration, they show a nodular, peripheral enhancement which, within 15–30 minutes, will be uniform and obscure the mass from the surrounding liver. T1W post-contrast MR sequences demonstrate the same 'centripetal' enhancement, but the lesion remains brighter than the surrounding liver. A further

characteristic MR feature of a hemangioma is that the lesions remain very bright on long T2W sequences. This has been termed the 'lightbulb' sign.

Hepatic adenoma

This mass occurs in younger women and has an association with the oral contraceptive pill. It is usually symptomatic (the patient has abdominal pain) and is the result of bleeding from within the adenoma. This bleeding and the presence of fat within the lesion have particular MR signal characteristics that allow the diagnosis to be made.

Focal nodular hyperplasia (FNH)

Often an asymptomatic incidental finding, FNH represents normal hepatocytes and Kupffer cells, arranged abnormally. An arteriovenous malformation may form the central nidus. Approximately 50% have a central scar. It is typically hypoechoic on ultrasound. MR characteristics are similar to the surrounding liver (unlike hepatic adenoma) on T1W and T2W sequences. The lesion typically enhances promptly on MR, but the scar characteristically shows delayed enhancement.

Hepatocellular carcinoma (HCC)

Hepatocellular carcinoma often occurs in association with underlying liver problems, e.g., viral hepatitis, cirrhosis or alcoholic liver disease. For this reason those with established cirrhosis should be enrolled in a hepatocellular carcinoma ultrasound surveillance program. A knowledge of the history and background imaging findings can be very helpful in making the diagnosis. Elevation of serum alpha-fetoprotein is characteristic, except in those with the fibrolamellar variant—younger patients with normal livers.

Hepatocellular carcinoma is solitary in 50% of cases, multifocal in 20%, and diffuse in 30%. A surrounding capsule, internal septa, daughter nodules, and tumor thrombus in adjacent veins are helpful diagnostic features.

On CT, the tumor is seen as a low attenuation mass within the liver. Arterial phase enhancement is seen, both on CT and MRI. Central areas of necrosis are characteristic. On nuclear medicine studies, uptake of gallium 67 (Ga^{67}) occurs within the mass, whereas with technetium^{99m} (Tc^{99m})

sulfur colloid, isotope is taken up by the surrounding liver, not the tumor.

Metastases

Occasionally, liver metastases can calcify, e.g., colloid colorectal metastases, and therefore can be identified on the abdominal radiograph. Usually, however, the diagnosis of metastatic disease requires cross-sectional imaging. On ultrasound, the appearances are of dark (hypoechoic) circular solid areas within the liver. On CT, these dark areas are of low attenuation. On MR, liver metastases are typically of lower signal on T1W, and of higher signal on T2W sequences, than the surrounding liver. A useful rule on MR is that the signal characteristics of liver metastatic lesions are the same as the spleen.

Hydatid disease

Plain films may show liver calcification, oval or circular being typical; ultrasound (and MR) will confirm the cystic nature of the lesion and the presence of daughter cysts. CT will localize the disease and define the extent.

Biliary diseases

Gallstones

See Chapter 4.

Cholangiocarcinoma

Cholangiocarcinoma is an adenocarcinoma that arises from bile duct epithelium. It is classified as intra- or extrahepatic. Intrahepatic cholangiocarcinomas are further differentiated by location into hilar (Klatskin tumors) or peripheral. Peripheral is defined as being distal to the second bifurcation of the left or right hepatic duct.

Peripheral cholangiocarcinoma

This is usually seen on CT and MR as a large, well-defined, lobular mass, with peripheral enhancement on both modalities.

Hilar cholangiocarcinoma (the Klatskin tumor)

Hilar cholangiocarcinoma represents more than 50% of large bile duct cancers. The most common presentation (> 70%) is as a small infiltrating tumor. Because of the location, jaundice is an early presenting feature. CT may demonstrate a thickened, high attenuation duct wall that occludes the lumen.

Extrahepatic cholangiocarcinoma

The cardinal feature on US, CT, and MR studies is the demonstration of biliary dilatation proximal to the lesion, and of normal caliber distal to it. The lesion itself can be located at the level of the bile duct's diameter transition. Contrast examinations, e.g., PTC or ERCP, will identify the level of the disease as a biliary stricture. Both techniques permit subsequent therapeutic intervention and cytological evaluation.

 Ulcerative colitis is a risk factor for the development of cholangiocarcinoma.

Bile duct strictures

Benign bile duct strictures are the result of trauma, surgery, ERCP, inflammatory processes, infections, and cholangitis, either primary sclerosing or Asiatic. US, CT, and MR (MRC) will confirm the biliary dilatation. MRC in particular is useful in determining the level of any stricture. Sclerosing cholangitis has a characteristic 'beaded' appearance of the biliary tree on MRC.

Pancreatic diseases

Pancreatic carcinoma

On both US and CT, pancreatic adenocarcinoma appears as a darker mass within the gland (see Fig. 22.7). CT delineates the lesion more effectively, can confirm biliary and/or pancreatic ductal dilatation, atrophy of the distal gland, tumor infiltration into the surrounding structures (particularly tumor involvement of the mesenteric and portal vessels), lymphadenopathy and metastatic spread. Both US and CT permit image-guided biopsy.

 If multiple hepatic cysts are seen, assess the kidneys for polycystic kidney disease.

 Beading of the biliary tree is characteristic of primary sclerosing cholangitis—check for a history of associated ulcerative colitis.

Case conference

 An 82-year-old man was referred to the hepatobiliary surgeons with a 3-month history of vague abdominal pain, anorexia and 5 kg weight loss. He had a past medical history of three myocardial infarctions and emphysema. On clinical examination he was noted to be jaundiced, and biochemical evaluation confirmed cholestatic jaundice. His CA 19-9 marker was noted to be significantly elevated.

Abdominal radiograph

The gas pattern is unremarkable. There is no evidence of intestinal obstruction or perforation.

Minor degenerative changes are noted in the lumbar vertebrae, but there is no evidence of metastatic disease.

Ultrasound of abdomen

The gallbladder is distended and no stones are visible. The common hepatic duct is significantly dilated at 1.4 cm. There is intrahepatic duct dilatation. Multiple hypoechoic lesions measuring approximately 1 cm are noted within the liver. The pancreas is obscured by gas. No other abnormality is seen.

CT chest and abdomen

In the chest there are multiple lesions seen within both lungs. The liver also contains multiple low attenuation lesions, and the biliary dilatation is confirmed. There is a 4 cm low attenuation mass in the head of the pancreas. Dilatation of the distal pancreatic duct and atrophy of the distal gland are also noted. The mass abuts the mesenteric vessels, with loss of the fat plane between them. The appearances are consistent with a pancreatic carcinoma with evidence of local invasion. There are liver and lung metastases.

In view of the advanced nature of the disease, and the patient's general health, palliation was performed by placing a biliary stent endoscopically at ERCP. Following this, the patient's jaundice resolved quickly. He was discharged to the care of his family, general practitioner, and palliative care team. He demised 6 weeks later.

6. Altered Bowel Habit/ Rectal Bleeding

Altered bowel habit is a common gastrointestinal presenting complaint. Feces containing blood, fresh or changed, is by definition, altered.

Imaging should be considered only after a full history and an appropriate assessment, including digital rectal examination (DRE). Not all patients will warrant radiological assistance for diagnosis—hemorrhoids and irritable bowel syndrome, for example, are clinical diagnoses (albeit the latter established by exclusion). However, at times imaging can reassure both the patient and clinician. Those that do justify further investigation may benefit from imaging in isolation or, more commonly, in conjunction with endoscopic studies. Consideration should be given to the urgency of the clinical presentation. An acute hospital admission with suspected small bowel obstruction will require immediate attention, whereas a chronic history of altered bowel habit may be undertaken as an outpatient with follow-up at clinic.

Plain AXRs are a sensible starting point for many patients, most importantly to exclude obstruction or perforation, and are frequently requested for non-specific abdominal pain. Following these, contrast studies are the next likely imaging step, although CT is increasingly used, including the technique of CT colonography.

The exclusion of colorectal carcinoma (CRC), diverticular, and inflammatory bowel disease (IBD) forms a substantial proportion of those patients presenting with altered bowel habit and rectal bleeding. Of course, these pathologies can coexist, making interpretation more of a challenge. In the case of CRC, ulcerative colitis (UC) and diverticular disease, a contrast enema is the imaging investigation of choice. For Crohn's disease, a small bowel series is more appropriate, as the terminal ileum is the most frequently affected area. A barium enema should be considered if there is suspicion of large bowel Crohn's disease.

Crohn's disease is asymmetrical and discontinuous; ulcerative colitis is symmetrical and continuous.

In a limited number of cases, more specialist imaging studies are useful. A radiolabel led white cell scan proves helpful in delineating the extent of inflamed or affected bowel in IBD. Those with persistent or significant rectal bleeding may benefit from a radiolabel led red cell scan or mesenteric angiography—most valuably in those bleeding acutely—to identify a focal source.

Angiodysplasia and irritable bowel syndrome are both diagnoses of exclusion.

Double contrast enema produces excellent large bowel mucosal detail.

A labelled red cell scan essentially requires active bleeding at the time of investigation.

Small bowel diseases

Crohn's disease
The plain abdominal x-ray may be unremarkable, but can show, on occasion, intestinal obstruction or

The features of Crohn's disease on contrast study include:

- Rose-thorn ulceration.
- Aphthoid ulcers.
- Cobblestoning.
- Strictures.
- Bowel loop separation.
- Pseudosacculations.
- Thickened valvulae conniventes.

Fig. 6.1 The features of Crohn's disease.

evidence of toxic megacolon. It is important to review the sacroiliac (SI) joints for evidence of sacroiliitis (see Ch. 9).

The hallmarks of Crohn's disease are that it is most common at the terminal ileum, is asymmetrical, and discontinuous. On small bowel barium studies, i.e., small bowel series or enema (enteroclysis), look for 'rose-thorn' and aphthoid ulcers, thickened blunted valvulae conniventes, cobblestoning, strictures ('string sign of Kantor;' see Fig. 21.14), bowel loop separation, and pseudosacculations. Large bowel features are similar (see Fig. 6.1).

Scleroderma

Scleroderma is a systemic disorder. Malabsorption may follow small bowel involvement. On barium studies, the bowel is hypomobile or atonic, and the lumen, diffusely enlarged, has thickened mucosal folds and pseudosacculations. It is said to have a 'hidebound' appearance. Similarly, the large bowel is atonic with pseudosacculations on the antimesenteric border.

Celiac disease

Barium examination demonstrates jejunal dilatation but normal fold thickness. The number of jejunal folds decreases and the ileal folds increase. This reversal ('flip-flop' pattern) occurs with chronic disease. On the small bowel barium examination there is segmentation of the barium. The 'moulage' sign—a wax cast appearance of barium in a featureless tube—is due to the complete effacement of the mucosal folds. Celiac disease may be complicated by lymphoma.

Large bowel diseases

Colorectal cancer

Plain abdominal radiographs may be normal in the absence of intestinal obstruction, in which case there is evidence typically of small bowel obstruction with right-sided tumors, and of large bowel obstruction with left-sided lesions.

In the well-prepared patient, double contrast barium enema (DCBE) should allow excellent visualization of the colorectal mucosa. All non-mobile filling defects must be viewed with suspicion, as colorectal cancers evolve from polyps (see Fig. 21.18). Radiologically, there are two chief forms of colorectal cancer on DCBE: 'apple-core' strictures (usually left-sided) and ulcerating or linear masses involving one wall of the bowel (usually right-sided; see Fig. 21.20).

Conditions predisposing to colorectal cancer include:
- Familial adenoma polyposis coli.
- Hereditary non-polyposis colorectal cancer.
- Gardner's syndrome (associated with osteomas of skull and mandible and desmoids of mesentery).
- Inflammatory bowel disease.

Approximately half of all colorectal cancers arise within 20 cm of the anal margin. As the sigmoid colon can be very tortuous, this, in the presence of diverticular disease—endemic in the over 60s—necessitates careful evaluation.

Familial polyposis coli is a genetically transmitted (autosomal dominant) colorectal carcinomatous disease which presents in the second or third decade of life. Radiological manifestations on DCBE are of thousands of polyps 'carpeting' the colonic mucosa (see Fig. 21.19). Associated disorders include Gardner's syndrome, in which polyposis is found with osteomas of the mandible. Like polyposis coli, it is autosomal dominant.

CT is the mainstay of staging and will exclude lymphadenopathy, liver metastatic disease, the presence of adjacent visceral involvement, such as that of the bladder and ureter, and the tumor itself. CT colonography is an imaging method gaining increased acceptance in the diagnosis of colorectal polyps. The patient, having taken a standard bowel preparation to cleanse the colon, undergoes standard bowel insufflation with a rectal catheter. CT of the abdomen and pelvis is performed in both the prone and supine positions. Polyps and masses, unlike fecal residue, should be fixed, regardless of patient positioning.

The role of MR is currently being evaluated as an imaging tool in rectal cancer. Unlike CT, the layers of the rectal wall can be delineated, and therefore local disease staging, particularly mesorectal involvement, can be performed and the need for adjuvant therapy evaluated. Some centers currently use endoanal ultrasound to evaluate the depth of tumor involvement in anorectal cancer.

CT colonography is particularly useful in infirm patients who are unable to undergo colonoscopy or barium enema.

In familial polyposis coli total colectomy with ileorectal anastomosis or ileostomy is usually undertaken before 20 years of age before carcinoma develops.

Colorectal cancers are glucose avid following [18]FDG (fluorodeoxyglucose) administration. PET imaging is therefore very useful in staging the tumor and quantitating tumor recurrence and metastatic disease.

Diverticular disease
See Chapter 4.

Ulcerative colitis
Important AXR findings are toxic megacolon, which is seen in $\leq 10\%$ of cases (see Fig. 21.25). Sacroiliitis may also be noted. The hallmark of this disease on contrast studies is that it is, unlike Crohn's disease, symmetrical and continuous, beginning at the rectum and progressing proximally (see Fig. 21.21). The rectum, however, can appear radiologically normal if the patient has been using steroid enemas. Mucosal ulcers, a granular mucosa, and thumbprinting are seen, as is blunting of the haustral folds and widening of the presacral space (> 2 cm on a single contrast enema). Inflammatory (pseudo) and filiform (daughter) polyps occur following attacks and in the quiescent phase, respectively. Strictures are rarer than in Crohn's disease and should be differentiated from carcinoma. The incidence of carcinoma rises dramatically in UC if extensive colitis has been present for more than 10 years. Typically patients are invited to enroll in an endoscopic surveillance program.

The rectum may appear normal on barium enema despite ulcerative colitis being an ascending disease. This is due to the use of steroid enemas.

Infections
Tuberculosis
Colonic tuberculosis (TB) classically affects the terminal ileum. On contrast studies, there is contraction of the cecal wall, upward retraction of the cecum and straightening of the ileocecal angle. Less than half of cases have pulmonary tuberculosis. TB of the small bowel produces localized areas of thickened, irregular, and distorted folds in non-dilated bowel.

Some infections involving the bowel can be conveniently categorized by specific radiological appearances:
- *Colonic 'polyps'*—amoebiasis and schistosomiasis, which usually involve the rectum and can be associated with strictures.
- *Colonic strictures*—schistosomiasis (rectosigmoid); amoebiasis (descending colon); chlamydia, which produces lymphogranuloma venereum (rectosigmoid), is long and tubular, and can undergo malignant change when chronic.
- *Megacolon*—salmonella and amoebiasis.

Angiodysplasia
Angiodysplasia is the result of blood vessel dilatation within the bowel wall, chiefly in the cecum and the ascending colon. This elusive diagnosis, a recognized cause of occult large bowel bleeding, classically (if rarely) manifests itself angiographically as small pools of contrast with early venous filling. Such angiographic lesions are

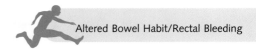

difficult to confirm by the surgeon or pathologist, but right hemicolectomy is often curative.

Hemorrhoids

A clinical diagnosis. No radiology required. However, this is an important clinical diagnosis to make to avoid unnecessary radiological investigation.

Intestinal obstruction

See Chapter 4.

Pseudomembranous colitis

Pseudomembranous colitis is related to the organism *Clostridium difficile* and antibiotic therapy, particularly clindamycin and third generation cephalosporins. The vast majority of uncomplicated cases are diagnosed by stool culture and treated accordingly without the need for imaging. Plain film

features include adynamic bowel, thumbprinting, and thickened haustra. The process tends to involve the whole colon. Ascites, small bowel dilatation with edema of the valvulae conniventes, and thickening and separation of the bowel loops are recognized associations. Differential diagnoses, radiologically, would include ischemic colitis and chronic inflammatory bowel disease.

Barium enema is contraindicated if the bowel is dilated with evidence of thumbprinting on plain film.

Paralytic ileus

See Chapter 4.

Case conferences

Case 1

A 58-year-old lady was admitted to the gastroenterology unit with a 2-month history of diarrhea. She admits to a 4 kg weight loss over the past 3 months. There were no other symptoms. On clinical and hematological examination she was noted to be anemic (microcytic hypochromic type). Her CEA was raised at 13.7. There were no other symptoms. Upper GI endoscopy and rigid sigmoidoscopy were normal.

Abdominal radiograph

The bowel gas pattern is normal with no evidence of mechanical obstruction or perforation. No other significant abnormality is seen.

Barium enema

Barium flows freely around the large bowel to the cecum and outlines the appendix. There is a filling defect on the

medial wall of the ascending colon which is a constant finding on multiple projections. The appearances are very suspicious of a carcinoma.

Small bowel series

The mucosal pattern of the jejunum and ileum is normal. The terminal ileum outlines normally. There is no evidence of stricturing, ulceration, or obstruction.

A colonoscopy was performed and this confirmed a mass lesion in the ascending colon. Multiple biopsies were taken and these confirmed the diagnosis of colonic carcinoma.

CT chest/abdomen/pelvis

A dynamically enhanced multidetector CT study was performed throughout the chest, abdomen, and pelvis.

Within the chest, there is no evidence of pulmonary metastases. No hilar or mediastinal lymphadenopathy is seen. On the abdominal images, the liver outlines normally with no evidence of metastases. There is no significant lymphadenopathy or ascites. There is an abnormal mass centered on the ascending colon. The surrounding fat planes are normal. No pelvic lesion is seen.

PET–CT
There is a glucose-avid lesion present within the right colon. The PET–CT location corresponds with that seen on the multidetector CT study. No other areas of increased uptake were identified within the chest, abdomen, or pelvis.

A right hemicolectomy was performed. The histological staging was Dukes B.

Case 2
An 82-year-old lady was admitted to hospital with a 3-day history of worsening lower abdominal pain. On examination she was noted to be pyrexial (39.2°C) and had a leucocytosis. She exhibited abdominal tenderness in the suprapubic and left iliac fossa regions. There was no significant past medical history.

Abdominal radiograph
The bowel gas pattern is normal. There is no evidence of intestinal obstruction or perforation.

Ultrasound
The gallbladder, biliary tree, liver, pancreas, and spleen outline normally. Both kidneys are sonographically normal. Within the pelvis there is a 6 cm fluid-filled mass seen separately from the bladder. The appearances are very suspicious of an abscess.

Contrast enema
An enema was performed with water-soluble contrast media. There is significant diverticular disease present with an associated stricture in the sigmoid colon. Scattered diverticula are noted elsewhere. No obstruction or extravasation is seen.

CT abdomen
The upper abdominal viscera are normal. In particular there is no evidence of liver metastases. Within the pelvis, there is a low attenuation mass adjacent to the sigmoid colon. The wall of this is noted to enhance. Sigmoid diverticula are also noted. The appearances are consistent with a pelvic abscess.

CT drainage
(The procedure, including the risks and benefits, were explained. Informed and written consent was obtained. The procedure was performed using an aseptic technique with local analgesia.)

The patient is in the supine position. A skin marker is placed over the site of the collection within the pelvis. The subsequent images demonstrate the local anesthetic needle in situ. A larger needle is then seen within the collection. A guide wire is placed through the needle and the needle withdrawn. Dilators are passed over the wire into the abscess, a 12F gauge drain is passed over the wire and placed on free drainage.

250 mL of purulent fluid was aspirated and the patient became apyrexial overnight.

Follow-up CT confirmed that the abscess had significantly reduced. It was agreed to resect the diseased strictured segment of sigmoid colon, and a Hartmann's procedure was performed (sigmoid colectomy and oversewing of the rectal stump, with end colostomy). It was anticipated that the colostomy could be reversed in the future and the left colon anastomosed to the rectum when the patient had fully recovered.

7. Scrotal or Groin Mass

The most common groin masses are hernias and the diagnosis is usually established on clinical examination. Occasionally imaging studies are required to confirm the diagnosis.

Radiological evaluation of the scrotum is usually performed with ultrasound, not only because of the accessible location, but also because of the gonads' radiosensitivity. The most common indication for scrotal ultrasound is to evaluate a mass; the most common diagnosis to exclude is testicular malignancy.

Scrotal mass

Primary testicular neoplasms

Testicular tumors are divided into germ cell and non-germ cell tumors.

Greater than 90% of tumors are germ cell and are typically malignant. Non-germ cell tumors are usually benign. Germ cell tumors are divided into seminomatous and non-seminomatous tumors. The most common of the latter group is teratoma.

Seminoma

The peak age for presentation of seminoma is the fourth and fifth decades. Although less aggressive than other testicular tumors, metastases are identified at presentation in 25%. On ultrasound, seminoma is characteristically a dark (hypoechoic) solid focal lesion confined within the tunica albuginea (see Fig. 22.19). Calcification and cystic change are rare.

Teratoma

Teratomas tend to be benign in childhood and malignant in adults. On ultrasound, unlike the uniformly hypoechoic seminoma, teratoma is heterogenous with cystic and calcific components.

Secondary malignancy

Lymphoma and leukemia are the most common secondary malignancies affecting the testis. Ultrasound appearances of both are non-specific, although lymphoma is bilateral in half of cases.

Testicular torsion

Testicular torsion is a clinical diagnosis. Although there is no arterial flow within the torted testis, Doppler ultrasound is currently considered unreliable as peripheral and intermittent flow patterns can still be identified in torsion and intermittent torsion, respectively. The diagnosis must therefore be based on the clinical presentation.

Hydrocele

Hydroceles are identified as anechoic (black) areas around the testis (see Fig. 22.18). Septations can be seen on occasion, and indicate chronicity.

The clinical diagnosis of a hydrocele should be followed up with ultrasound because of the association between hydrocele and testicular malignancy.

Varicocele

A varicocele is a collection of veins around the testis. On Doppler ultrasound, flow can be identified within these vessels, particularly if, while scanning, the patient is asked to increase their intra-abdominal pressure (Valsalva maneuver) (see Fig. 22.20). Because the left testicular vein drains into the left renal vein, its obstruction by, for example, a renal cell carcinoma is a recognized association. Therefore, a left-sided varicocele should prompt inspection of the left kidney to exclude a mass lesion. As the right renal vein drains separately into the IVC, the association does not exist on that side.

Epididymal cysts

The epididymis sits on the posterolateral aspect of the testis, with its head perched on the superior testicular aspect. Cysts are identified as anechoic, echo-free lesions within the epididymal head (see Fig. 22.17). They are a frequent incidental finding in testicular ultrasound and are of no significance. They are not premalignant.

Testicular microlithiasis

Testicular microlithiasis is the presence of myriad tiny calcifications (1–3 mm) within the testis. Their etiology is obscure. There is some evidence that there is an association with testicular malignancy, so annual surveillance in these patients is currently recommended.

Inguinal/thigh mass

Hernia

The diagnosis of inguinal hernia is clinical. Unless the hernia contains fluid-filled structures such as small bowel it can be very difficult to appreciate on ultrasound. On occasion, CT or MR is employed when there is diagnostic difficulty. These will show the hernial defect and can identify which structures, if any, are within it. Rarely, herniography—a procedure where contrast is injected directly into the peritoneum, and the patient placed in various positions—is used to outline inguinal hernial sacs. Although this is invasive, it is particularly useful in confirming hernial recurrence.

Saphena varix

Saphena varix is a dilatation of the long saphenous vein, usually at the saphenofemoral junction. It is readily seen on ultrasound, and Doppler ultrasound will show flow and confirm if there is valvular incompetence within the system. It is seen in association with venous insufficiency.

Lymphadenopathy

Lymph nodes are a very common incidental finding on groin ultrasound. They are seen as small, solid, oval masses. As a rule, benign nodes are elliptical and usually have a fatty (bright) center on ultrasound. Replacement of this by darker, necrotic material—particularly if the nodes are significantly enlarged, circular and matted together—is suspicious of malignant infiltration (Fig. 7.1).

Femoral artery aneurysm

Aneurysms are pathologically enlarged arteries with non-parallel walls. The size, location, presence of flow, and thrombus can be determined with ultrasound. Femoral artery aneurysms are rare.

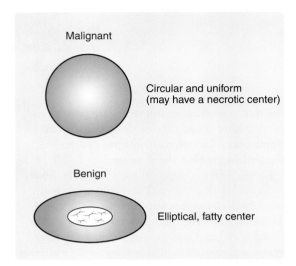

Fig. 7.1 Distinguishing the cause of lymphadenopathy.

Pseudoaneurysm

This is the name given to abnormal flow and distension within the vessel wall. This is a rare spontaneous event at the groin. However, following interventional procedures such as coronary artery catheterization via a groin puncture, leaking of blood can occur around the artery. This is generally known as a pseudoaneurysm, but is a misnomer. Doppler ultrasound can identify the collection, confirm that there is flow within it and can be used to accurately tamponade the hole. Ultrasound can also be used to guide percutaneous thrombin injection into the collection to thrombose the sac.

Ectopic/undescended testicle

Ultrasound can confirm absence of the testis within the scrotum and can localize testicular material within the inguinal canal. However, it is not effective at locating intra-abdominal testes. CT, and latterly MR, have been employed to identify ectopic testes. MR is preferred because there is no associated radiation (the patient group is generally young) and viable testicular material is bright on T2 weighted sequences (see Part II, Principles of Radiology), making it relatively easy to identify.

 If a femoral aneurysm is detected, look elsewhere for associated abdominal aortic or popliteal aneurysms.

Case conference

A 71-year-old man was admitted to the coronary care unit with severe central chest pain associated with nausea and sweating. ECG demonstrated elevated ST segments in the anterior chest leads consistent with an acute myocardial infarction. Lysis was contraindicated due to a recent hemorrhagic stroke. The decision was made for rescue percutaneous coronary angioplasty (PCA).

The management plan was discussed with the patient as were the risks and benefits of intervention, the patient agreed to coronary stenting if suitable. Coronary angiography confirmed the presence of a high-grade stenosis of the left anterior descending coronary artery. The procedure was technically routine. The following day, it was noted that there was a prominent swelling at the puncture site, with surrounding bruising.

Ultrasound of right groin
The right common, superficial, and profunda femoral arteries are identified and are normal. There is good flow in all three vessels. Superficial to the right common femoral vessel there is a cystic collection which measures 1.8 cm. On Doppler imaging, there is active blood flow within it. Furthermore, a jet of blood is seen to emanate from the right common femoral artery into the collection. The appearances are consistent with active extravasation and a 'false aneurysm.'

A trial of compression was undertaken, but repeat ultrasound did not show any interval change. Discussion with the interventional radiologists led to ultrasound-guided percutaneous thrombin injection, which thrombosed the collection successfully.

He was discharged the following week with review arrangements and a number of new medications.

Back pain is a very common presenting complaint. The differential diagnosis of the underlying cause is wide, but the most common cause is mechanical back pain. Classically, plain radiographs have been the mainstay for the imaging of back pain, although it is clear that they are relatively insensitive in excluding significant discovertebral degeneration. MR is the investigation of choice.

Summary of causes
- Degenerative diseases.
- Inflammatory diseases.
- Infection.
- Neoplastic.
- Metabolic.

Degenerative diseases

Disc disease
On the plain lumbar spine radiograph, the characteristic findings of degeneration are narrowing of the intervertebral disc space, sclerosis of the adjacent vertebral bodies, and osteophyte formation. On MR imaging, the degenerate, dehydrated disc, unlike the normally hydrated (bright, high signal) disc, appears dark on the T2 weighted (T2W) sequence. This is because it has become dehydrated. Altered signal may be seen in the adjacent vertebral end plates. These zones of altered signal are called 'Modic' changes and help the radiologist determine the chronicity of the degeneration.

It is important to remember that 30% of asymptomatic 30 year olds and almost 100% of 60 year olds will have evidence of disc degeneration on MR. It is crucial therefore to ensure that the radiological findings are consistent with the clinical presentation.

Inflammatory diseases

Seronegative arthropathy
Seronegative arthropathies that affect the vertebral column include psoriasis, enteropathic arthropathies (e.g., ulcerative colitis, Crohn's disease, and Whipple's disease), ankylosing spondylitis, and Reiter's syndrome (mnemonic: PEAR).

Ankylosing spondylitis
Ankylosing spondylitis primarily affects the axial skeleton (spine, pelvis, hip, and shoulder girdle). It typically begins in the sacroiliac joints (see Fig. 23.12b) and goes on to affect the spine. Features on the spinal radiograph include calcification of the annulus fibrosis (syndesmophytes), the 'shiny corner' and 'square vertebra' signs, produced by erosion of the corners of the vertebral bodies and calcification of the anterior longitudinal ligament. Syndesmophytes flowing across several vertebral bodies produce the classical 'bamboo spine' appearance (see Fig. 23.12a).

Enteropathic arthropathy
Conditions such as ulcerative colitis, Crohn's disease, and Whipple's disease produce spondylitic changes as in ankylosing spondylitis. The sacroiliac inflammatory changes, as in ankylosing spondylitis, are bilateral and symmetrical.

Psoriatic arthropathy
Like ankylosing spondylitis, the spinal manifestation of this condition is with syndesmophytes and sacroiliitis. The sacroiliitis progresses to bony fusion less commonly than in ankylosing spondylitis, and is unilateral or asymmetrical in just less than half of cases.

Reiter's syndrome
See Chapter 9.

Neoplastic spinal disease

As with neoplasms elsewhere, secondary metastatic deposits are more common than primary bone tumors.

Primary bone tumors
Benign tumors
Benign tumors of the vertebral body include hemangioma, aneurysmal bone cyst, giant cell

* Absent pedicle on this vertebra

Fig. 8.1 Vertebral spinous metastasis.

tumor, osteoid osteoma, and osteoblastoma (mnemonic: HAG O2). Osteoblastoma occurs in the posterior elements of the vertebral body and is expansile with a 'soap-bubble' appearance; 50% have calcifications. Osteoid osteoma is usually located within cortical bone and is seen as a sclerotic lesion with a central lucency—the nidus. The classic history is of bone pain, worse at night, and relieved by aspirin.

Malignant tumors
Myeloma and plasmacytoma
On plain films, myeloma looks osteopenic, but has different spinal appearances on CT in its acute and chronic phases. Acutely, there are multiple holes (this has been likened to a 'Swiss cheese'), and chronically trabecular thickening that mimics Paget's disease (see Fig. 23.5). Plasmacytoma is a focal presentation of myeloma. Although it can manifest itself in a variety of ways, the classic appearance on lumbar spine radiograph is of an expansile or destructive lucent lesion. In addition, the appearance of myeloma in the skull is known as 'salt and pepper skull'.

Chordoma
Chordoma is derived from notochordal remnants. 90% of cases occur in two locations, both midline: the clivus (basisphenoid) at the top of the spine, and the sacrum at the bottom. On plain x-rays there is bone destruction and there may be an appreciable soft tissue mass. CT and MR will demonstrate the degree of bone destruction, involvement of adjacent structures and the soft tissue mass.

Secondary bone tumors
On spinal radiographs, metastatic involvement manifests itself as either osteoblastic (bone forming—looks sclerotic; see Fig. 23.11) or osteoclastic (bone resorbing—looks lytic; see Fig. 23.11). Classically, the pedicles are involved and, on the anterior view, this absent pedicle has been likened to an eye winking (the visible 'eye' representing the normal pedicle and the closed eye, the metastatic deposit; Fig. 8.1). Metastatic disease does not generally traverse the intervertebral discs (unlike osteomyelitis, which typically does).

It is sometimes possible to suggest the primary location of the cancer by the appearance: sclerotic lesions (bright, bone-forming) occur with prostatic cancer, carcinoid, and lymphoma; lytic disease (dark, bone-losing) is associated with breast and bronchus, and lytic, expansile lesions with the kidney, thyroid, myeloma, and melanoma. MRI elegantly demonstrates metastatic disease and also complications such as spinal cord compression (see Fig. 23.14b,c).

Metastatic disease does not generally traverse the intervertebral discs, unlike osteomyelitis.

Metabolic bone disease

Common etiologies would include:
- Osteoporosis.
- Osteomalacia.
- Rickets.
- Hyperparathyroidism (primary and secondary).
- Acromegaly.

Osteoporosis

Osteoporosis is defined as a reduction of normal quality bone. On spinal x-rays, there is accentuation of the primary (vertical) trabeculae, resorption of the secondary (horizontal) trabeculae, and reduced bone density (osteopenia).

These weakened vertebrae are therefore vulnerable and can collapse. This is typically manifest as an anterior wedge fracture or a 'codfish' biconcave collapse. 'Insufficiency'

fractures are also seen at the symphysis pubis, femoral neck, pubic rami, and sacrum.

The reduction of bone density can be calculated by CT bone density programs or more usually by dual energy x-ray absorptiometry (DEXA) scan (Fig. 8.2). The score produced measures bone density against healthy bone (T score). A T score between –1.0 and –2.5 represents osteopenia, and less than –2.5, osteoporosis. The 'T' score represents an average

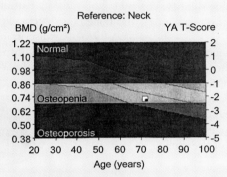

Region	BMD [1] (g/cm²)	Young-Adult [2] T-Score	Age-Matched [3] Z-Score
Neck	0.721	-2.2	-0.4
Wards	0.526	-3.0	-0.7
Troch	0.746	-0.4	0.7
Shaft	0.987	-	-
Total	0.832	-1.4	0.1

Region	BMD [1] (g/cm²)	Young-Adult [2] T-Score	Age-Matched [3] Z-Score
L1	0.812	-2.7	-0.8
L2	0.814	-3.2	-1.4
L3	0.836	-3.0	-1.2
L4	0.846	-3.0	-1.1
L2-L4	0.833	-3.1	-1.2

Fig. 8.2 Bone densitometry results for (a) osteopenic hip, (b) osteoporotic spine.

score for gender; the 'Z' score is age and gender matched.

In the elderly patient with ongoing hip discomfort following a fall, consider an insufficiency fracture of the pelvis.

Osteomalacia

This is defined as increased uncalcified osteoid in the mature skeleton. Radiographic manifestations include reduction in bone density, coarsening of the trabecular pattern, Looser's zones, and bone softening.

Looser's zones (or pseudofractures) represent focal osteoid collections and are seen perpendicular to the long axis of bones. Common sites include the femoral necks, pubic rami, and long bones. Bone softening manifests as biconcave vertebral bodies and elsewhere as bowing of the long bones, 'protrusio acetabulae' and basilar invagination of the skull.

Rickets

Rickets is defined as increased uncalcified osteoid in the immature skeleton due to vitamin D deficiency (see Fig. 23.8).

Delayed bone maturation and growth results, but radiographic reduction in bone density is not common. The bone, as in osteomalacia, is softened, and the radiological manifestations generally result from this. In the spine, the vertebrae become biconcave.

Hyperparathyroidism

See Chapter 9.

Acromegaly

Acromegaly is the result of excessive growth hormone's action on the mature skeleton. On plain radiographs, there is an increased sagittal diameter of the chest with an associated kyphosis. The vertebral bodies demonstrate increased anterior and transverse dimensions with 'posterior scalloping' (see also Ch. 9).

Paget's disease

Paget's disease has three phases: lytic, mixed, and sclerotic. In the lumbar spine, features include coarsening of the trabeculae and cortices. Pelvic involvement is frequent and coarsening of the iliopectineal line is classic.

Pathological fractures and spinal stenosis may occur. Pelvic Paget's disease may be difficult to discriminate from osteoblastic metastases, but the diagnostic clue is that Paget's disease always begins at a bone end. Metastases occur randomly.

Carefully correlate the pattern of clinical joint disease and bone profile blood results with radiographic appearances.

Isotope bone scans are relatively insensitive to the diagnosis of multiple myeloma because of their lack of osteoblastic activity.

Pelvic Paget's disease can be distinguished from osteoblastic metastases as Paget's disease begins at the bone edge, metastases are random.

Case conference

A 48-year-old bricklayer was reviewed at the orthopedic outpatient clinic. He complained of a 6-week history of severe lower back pain. For the last 2 weeks, the pain had radiated down the left leg to the great toe and was refractory to a number of medications prescribed by the on-call GP service.

On examination his straight leg raising was reduced to 30° on the left, but was normal on the right. The left ankle jerk was also noted to be absent. There was no evidence of any 'red flag' signs.

Lumbar spine radiograph
There is loss of the lumbar lordosis. There is reduction of the L5/S1 disc space with osteophyte formation. There is no evidence of a fracture or vertebral infiltration.

MR lumbar spine
Sagittal T1W, T2W, and axial T2W sequences were performed. There is loss of hydration of the lower three lumbar intervertebral disc spaces. There is loss of height of the L5/S1 disc with a posterior disc bulge. On the axial images there is a posterior disc protrusion centrally and towards the left lateral recess. There is significant effacement of the left side of the thecal sac and the prolapsed disc lies adjacent to the left S1 nerve root.

The radiologist informs the orthopedic team who arranges a clinically suitable date for surgery.

9. Joint Pain

Joint pain causes significant physical and functional burden. Despite great technical strides in nuclear medicine, ultrasound, CT, and MRI, plain radiographs remain the mainstay of clinical imaging.

Frequently plain radiographs are requested initially, but the yield of significant findings may be limited in relation to clinical symptoms. Further imaging should be tailored to the most likely diagnoses:

- Rheumatoid arthritis.
- Seronegative arthritis.
- Degenerative.
- Hemophilia.
- Metabolic.
- Infectious.
- Systemic.

Rheumatoid arthritis

Rheumatoid arthritis (RA) is a multisystem autoimmune disorder, where a symmetrical synovial and cartilaginous joint pathology is a variable component of systemic disease. The appendicular joints affected include those of the hands, feet, wrists, knees, ankles, elbows, hips, and shoulders. The axial skeleton may also be affected, i.e., the atlantoaxial and apophyseal joints.

The hand

On hand radiographs, RA tends to affect the metacarpophalangeal (MCP), proximal interphalangeal (PIP) and the intercarpal joints. In the wrist, the ulnar styloid and distal radioulnar joints are affected. The disease tends to affect the proximal portion of the joint surface more severely than the distal (see Fig. 23.21).

Initially there are joint effusions with synovial thickening, periarticular edema and osteoporosis. The changes are symmetrical. This is followed by joint space narrowing and erosion at the joint margins. In complicated cases, subluxation and malalignment of joints is seen with ulnar deviation, swan-neck and boutonnière deformity of the fingers, and ankylosis (fusion).

Rheumatoid arthritis affects the MCP and PIP joints; osteoarthritis typically affects the distal interphalangeal (DIP) joints.

Atlantoaxial joint

The cervical region of the spine is most commonly affected. Pathological change in the transverse atlantoaxial ligament (either laxity or ligament rupture) produces subluxation of the joint (Fig. 9.1). In 25% of severe RA patients, atlantoaxial subluxation can be demonstrated on flexion and extension lateral cervical spine radiographs. The distance between the posterior aspect of the anterior arch of the atlas and the dens should not exceed 3 mm in the adult. A wider space or one that changes between flexion and extension indicates subluxation. Radiographs of the atlantoaxial joint may also show erosions of the odontoid peg. Subluxation may affect other cervical levels, particularly C4/C5.

The hip and knee

The characteristic differentiation between rheumatoid and osteoarthritis (OA) at these joints is the uniform reduction in joint space seen in RA. OA has a more asymmetrical joint space involvement, affecting the superior aspect of the acetabular joint space at the hip and the medial compartment space of the knee. OA also tends to have more periarticular sclerotic change.

Seronegative arthritis

Psoriasis

Psoriatic arthropathy occurs in 5% of patients with psoriasis. The relationship with skin disease is variable. There are several arthropathic patterns in psoriasis: the most common is single joint involvement; others include a rheumatoid arthritis

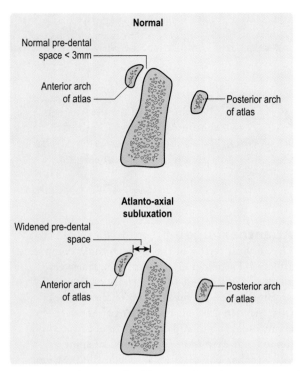

Fig. 9.1 Atlanto-axial subluxation (lateral projection).

type appearance, an arthritis affecting the DIP joints, a spinal distribution, and finally an arthritis mutilans.

Types of psoriatic arthropathy include:
- Mono/oligoarthritis.
- Ankylosing spondylitis.
- DIP predominance.
- Arthritis mutilans.
- Rheumatoid distribution.

Hands and feet
Soft tissue swelling is prominent, and involvement of a whole finger is known as a dactylitis ('sausage digit'). The arthropathy, which is asymmetric, is destructive and affects the DIP joints, with erosions beginning peripherally at the joint margins and advancing centrally ('cup and pencil' deformity). Tuft resorption may also be seen (see Fig. 23.17). A fine 'whiskering' can also be seen at the attachments of ligaments and tendons (the entheses). Bone density is normal.

Spine and sacroiliac joints
The sacroiliac changes are similar to those of ankylosing spondylitis, being symmetrical and bilateral. The spinal appearances (spondylitis),

however, are characteristically asymmetrical. Paravertebral ossification is a characteristic feature. Any spinal level may be affected.

Reiter's syndrome
This predominantly male disease is usually the sequela of sexually transmitted disease or dysentery and describes the association of urethritis, arthritis, eye and skin lesions. The arthropathy of Reiter's syndrome affects the feet and hands, the spine and the sacroiliac (SI) joints. X-ray appearances in the hands and feet are similar to psoriasis, with the foot more commonly affected than the hand. Calcaneal 'spurs' are a feature. SI joint appearances are similar to ankylosing spondylitis and psoriasis, with the spondylitic changes indistinguishable from psoriasis.

Ankylosing spondylitis
Ankylosing spondylitis usually affects young people. The disease, although it may affect large and even small joints, typically presents in the spine and sacroiliac joints. The presence of extra-axial disease is important as it alters clinical management (see Ch. 8).

Enteropathy
Patients with ulcerative colitis, Crohn's disease, and Whipple's disease can suffer from spinal and sacroiliac arthropathies similar to those seen in ankylosing spondylitis. Peripheral joint involvement is rarer, and features include loss of bone density, soft tissue swelling and synovitis. These changes reflect exacerbations of the disease—the peripheral arthropathy resolves as the disease remits, the spinal pathology does not.

Degenerative arthritis

Osteoarthritis
Osteoarthritis may be primary (polyarticular) or secondary (monoarticular). In the hands, the first carpal, metacarpal, and intercarpal joints are affected. In the feet the first metatarsophalangeal joint is affected. Osteophytes, sclerosis, and geodes (subchondral cysts) are characteristic, as is non-uniform joint narrowing and an asymmetrical distribution (see Figs 23.15, 23.23, 23.24; see also Ch. 8).

Radiographic features of osteoarthritis are illustrated in Figure 9.2.

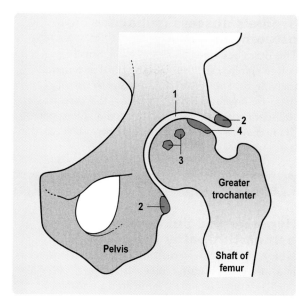

Fig. 9.2 Osteoarthritic changes at the hip: 1. Narrowed joint space; 2. osteophytes; 3. bone cysts; 4. subchondral sclerosis.

Hemophilia

Hemosiderin from a hemarthrosis is absorbed by synovium, which consequently becomes enlarged and prone to injury. This injury causes bleeding, more hemosiderin production, and further synovial enlargement. Hemorrhage also produces articular cartilage changes.

Radiographic features include joint effusions and epiphyseal enlargement secondary to hyperemic osteopenia. In the knee, there is epiphyseal enlargement, widening of the intercondylar notch and squaring of the inferior aspect of the patella. Subchondral cysts and joint space narrowing are also seen. At the ankle joint, tibiotalar slant is seen, secondary to narrowing of the lateral aspect of the distal tibial epiphysis. The 'hemophilic pseudotumor' may be seen in the pelvis. This manifests as an expansile lucent area within bone, usually the ilium.

Metabolic disorders

Gout

Gout results from hyperuricemia and presents with recurrent acute arthritis. In the acute phase, gout usually affects only one joint—often the first metatarsophalangeal joint of the foot (podagra). This manifests as soft tissue swelling, joint effusions, and loss of bone density around the joint. Chronically (chronic tophaceous gout), non-calcified nodules of calcium urate (tophi) adjacent to the joint are identified. Erosions, round or oval, lie in the long axis of the bone, pointing away from the joint (see Fig. 23.13). Intraosseous tophi—small cysts within the bone—are also seen. Bone density is normal. Diagnosis is by detection of negatively birefringent crystals from a joint aspirate.

 With an acute, red, hot, painful, swollen joint, septic arthritis should be excluded by joint aspiration.

Calcium pyrophosphate dehydrate (CPPD) deposition disease

CPPD is the commonest cause of an acutely swollen joint in the over 60-year-old age group.

CPPD deposition disease is the association of pseudogout, chondrocalcinosis, and an arthropathy. Pseudogout indicates a crystal synovitis that causes an acute inflammatory arthritis. Radiological findings in pseudogout are of joint effusions and soft tissue edema. Chondrocalcinosis is not a specific disease, but a radiological sign meaning the identification of joint crystals on x-ray. These can be CPPD or hydroxyapatite crystals. Hydroxyapatite crystal deposition is associated with hyperparathyroidism and milk–alkali syndrome.

In chronic CPPD arthropathy, features include subchondral cysts, articular surface breakdown and intra-articular fragments. Typical sites include the patellofemoral, elbow, radiocarpal, and MCP joints. Chondrocalcinosis, if present, tends to be seen in large joints like the shoulder, the hip, and the knee. The destructive arthropathy can mimic neuropathic joints (a pseudoneuropathy), but neurological examination is normal.

 Gout (uric acid) and pseudogout (CPPD) can be distinguished by the birefringence pattern of the crystals in the aspirated joint fluid.

Hemochromatosis

The arthropathy in hemochromatosis is due to the deposition of iron in the articular cartilage. Radiologically, the changes resemble CPPD with a predilection for the MCP joints of the second and third metacarpals, the midcarpals, and the carpometacarpal joints, with beak or hook-like osteophytes. Chondrocalcinosis is frequent.

Brodie's abscess (subacute osteomyelitis)

This describes a local bone infection, usually seen before epiphyseal closure, in the tibial or femoral metaphysis. *Staphylococcus aureus* is the usual causative organism. On plain x-rays, this is seen as a well-defined lucent lesion at the end of a long bone. There may be marginal sclerosis or periosteal reaction.

Infectious diseases

Osteomyelitis

Conventional radiographs are relatively insensitive in osteomyelitis. Up to 50% of bone has to be resorbed before bone destruction is visible, and x-ray changes can lag significantly behind clinical findings. Radiographic findings include soft tissue swelling, periosteal reaction, osteoporosis, reactive sclerosis, sequestrum, involucrum, soft tissue abscesses, and sinus tract formation. Bone scans are positive within hours of the onset of symptoms. A focal hotspot is the most common finding. On MRI the inflammation is seen to cause decreased signal on T1 weighted (T1W) and increased signal on T2W sequences. Good delineation of the extent of the disease—especially bone marrow, periosteal and surrounding soft tissue structures—is possible. MRI is more sensitive in the acute/subacute than the chronic phase.

Systemic diseases

Hypertrophic pulmonary osteoarthropathy (HPOA)

HPOA describes specific bony manifestations seen in a variety of systemic illnesses. These manifestations include a laminated periosteal reaction which affects the distal radius, ulna, tibia, and fibula. It is associated with finger clubbing and the etiology is given by the mnemonic 'CLUBBING:'

C   Cyanotic heart disease
L   Liver cirrhosis
U   Ulcerative colitis and Crohn's disease
B   Bronchiectasis (and other purulent lung disease such as empyema and abscess)
B   Bacterial endocarditis
I   Idiopathic
NG New growth (neoplasm).

Case conference

A 37-year-old medical secretary presents with a 6-month history of discomfort in the small joints of the hands. In particular she had found it especially troublesome removing her rings. She has a past medical history of pernicious anemia, diagnosed 10 years ago. The joints were particularly stiff in the mornings but improve after 2 hours of use. On examination there was evidence of active synovitis at the MCP and PIP joints.

She was commenced on non-steroidal anti-inflammatory drugs (NSAIDs) with good effect while awaiting results of blood tests and radiographs of the hands.

Radiograph of hands
The bones are osteopenic. There are erosive changes bilaterally at the MCP and PIP joints. Ulnar deviation of the phalanges is noted. The appearances are consistent with rheumatoid arthritis.

She was commenced on methotrexate, 10 mg weekly. Over the following 7 years she tried several disease-modifying anti-rheumatic drugs (DMARDs) with variable benefit before starting adalimumab therapy. At routine review she complained of increasing dyspnea and a dry cough.

Chest radiograph

The cardiac contour and pulmonary vascularity are normal. There are reticulonodular shadows present in both lungs, chiefly in the mid and lower zones. No focal mass lesion is evident. The appearances are consistent with interstitial lung disease.

Pulmonary function tests demonstrated a restrictive abnormality and a transfer factor of 48%. High resolution CT was performed.

High resolution CT of the chest

There are subpleural interstitial changes present in both lungs, chiefly in the lower zones. No focal mass is identified. There is no endobronchial mass or significant lymphadenopathy. The appearances are consistent with a linear non-septal pattern of interstitial lung disease. The history of methotrexate therapy and rheumatoid arthritis is noted, and the appearances would be in keeping with either of these. The differential diagnosis for these appearances would include amiodarone therapy, fibrosing alveolitis, asbestos-related lung disease and other connective tissue diseases.

Her rheumatologist discontinued her methotrexate and made arrangements for follow-up under the care of the respiratory physicians.

10. Neck Mass

Neck masses have been historically divided into midline, anterior and posterior triangle masses. Latterly, anatomical localization by disease level (the Sloane–Kettering Level I–VI classification) has gained widespread acceptance among head and neck surgeons. Ultrasound is very valuable for the evaluation of neck masses due to their relatively superficial location. Biopsy of the mass can be undertaken at this stage. Further characterization and staging is performed with a combination of CT, MR, and PET scanning.

Summary of causes
- Thyroid masses.
- Salivary diseases.
- Lymphadenopathy.
- Congenital/developmental.
- Miscellaneous.

Thyroid masses

Single nodule
Approximately 5% of the adult population have a thyroid nodule. Greater than 85–90% of thyroid nodules are benign and, if less than 1.5 cm in size, are likely to be occult (i.e., an incidental imaging finding).

A single nodule is the commonest nodular disease of the thyroid (80% of cases). Cystic change occurs in the majority of individuals (see Fig. 24.22). The presence of solid masses within the cyst, a size greater than 1 cm or the presence of microcalcification merits fine needle aspiration (FNA) to exclude cystic papillary carcinoma.

Indications for FNA of a thyroid nodule include:
- Solid mass within the cyst.
- Size > 1 cm.
- Microcalcification.

Adenomas
These account for 10% of thyroid nodular disease and are focal gland proliferations. They have a capsule which is demonstrated as the 'halo' sign on ultrasound. The distinction between follicular adenoma and carcinoma requires histology, but the demonstration of follicular cells on cytology represents an indication for surgical resection. When follicular neoplasms are resected, 80% are benign and 20% malignant.

Evidence of papillary cells is strongly correlated with malignancy.

Hyperfunctioning nodules
These may be hyperplastic or adenomas and have no specific sonographic characteristics.

Papillary carcinoma
This is the most common malignancy of the thyroid gland, accounting for two-thirds of thyroid malignancy. On ultrasound, these are seen as hypoechoic masses with a surrounding capsule. Microcalcifications are often present. The tumor is hypervascular on Doppler US. Fifty percent of patients have local nodal involvement at presentation. The finding of papillary cells on FNA is strongly correlated with malignancy as in practice they rarely represent an adenoma. The surgical procedure of choice, when papillary carcinoma is diagnosed, is total thyroidectomy.

Follicular carcinoma
This accounts for 20% of thyroid carcinomas and is associated with hyperplastic or adenomatous nodules in two-thirds of cases. There are no specific sonographic features but a thickened capsule and 'chaotic' vessels on Doppler ultrasound are described. The finding of follicular cells on FNA is an indication for surgery. Eighty percent of cases are benign and 20% malignant. The surgical

procedure of choice for a follicular mass is a hemithyroidectomy, with resection of the affected lobe and the isthmus. If malignant, completion thyroidectomy should be considered.

Anaplastic carcinoma

On ultrasound, this is hypoechoic, with areas of necrosis, amorphous calcification and local invasion. Anaplastic carcinoma has the worst prognosis. Overall, the most accurate sign of malignancy on ultrasound is microcalcification.

For the role of nuclear medicine in the thyroid nodule and in the parathyroid, see Part II.

Salivary diseases

Parotid adenoma

Parotid adenoma (also known as pleomorphic adenoma or benign mixed tumor of the parotid) is the most common mass of the parotid space (80%), occurring more commonly in females than in males, typically in the age range 30–60 years. The CT/MR appearances are those of a well-circumscribed, mildly enhancing mass (see Fig. 24.23). Cross-sectional imaging allows delineation of the mass relative to the facial nerve (i.e., within the superficial or deep lobe of the parotid).

Warthin's tumor (adenolymphoma)

This benign tumor is more commonly seen in males (> 60 years) and has a strong association with smoking. The tumor occurs typically in the parotid tail. It is usually inhomogeneous on CT/MR, with cystic areas and foci of hemorrhage. Mild contrast enhancement occurs. There is also increased uptake of fluorodeoxyglucose on PET scanning.

Parotid carcinoma

There are two tumor types: mucoepidermoid (60%) and adenoid cystic carcinoma. The role of cross-sectional imaging is to:
1. Confirm that the lesion is within the parotid.
2. Locate it either within the deep or the superficial lobe.

Radiologically, parotid carcinoma is an invasive intraparotid mass which enhances with contrast. Clinically, the mass is painful, and an association with facial nerve palsy is characteristic.

Sjögren's syndrome

Sjögren's syndrome is a chronic autoimmune disease which may be primary or secondary. Destruction of the lacrimal glands is a recognized feature. The imaging findings will depend on the stage of the disease. In the early stages on cross-sectional imaging, there are bilateral small cystic areas. Later, there are larger cysts (see Fig. 24.24) and solid lymphocytic masses with parenchymal destruction. Punctate calcification is also a feature. Sjögren's syndrome can be complicated by non-Hodgkin's lymphoma.

Lymphadenopathy

The most important question in the clinical imaging of lymph nodes is to separate reactive (benign) nodes from metastatic malignant nodes. This can prove challenging. Size is not an absolute criterion, but neck nodes greater than 1.5 cm are viewed with suspicion. In addition, persistent nodes identified in the posterior triangle of the neck represent cause for concern. Benign nodes tend to be elliptical, whereas malignant nodes are circular. The fatty center of benign nodes is replaced by hypoechoic necrotic tissue in malignancy. PET scanning is playing an increasing clinical role in determining reactive from malignant cervical lymphadenopathy.

Congenital/developmental diseases

Thyroglossal (duct) cyst

Thyroglossal duct cyst is the most common congenital neck lesion. It arises from the thyroglossal duct, which lies between the tongue's foramen cecum (superiorly) and the thyroid bed (inferiorly). It is classically a painless, mobile, midline swelling, but the site can be more lateral, inferiorly. It usually presents in the first decade, although 10% are seen in the third and fourth decades.

On ultrasound, it is anechoic. CT demonstrates a low attenuation mass and, on MRI, cystic composition (low signal T1 weighted, high signal T2 weighted).

The presence of a solid mass or calcification should raise suspicion of a complicating papillary carcinoma of the thyroid (rare, less than 1%).

Branchial cyst

This cyst develops from the second branchial cleft and occurs in teenagers and young adults. Branchial cysts are significantly more common in males. The most common of branchial anomalies (95%), it presents as a mass at the anterior aspect of the sternomastoid muscle, typically the upper third. On ultrasound, CT, and MR it is cystic with non-enhancing walls unless infected. It contains variable quantities of protein which produce a spectrum of signals on MR imaging.

Cystic hygroma

Cystic hygroma (also known as lymphangioma) is composed of dilated lymphatic spaces, usually presents at birth and early childhood, and has an association with Turner's syndrome. It is multiloculated and characteristically insinuates itself between neck structures, but without any significant mass effect. On ultrasound, CT, and MR the appearances are those of a cystic lesion. Hemorrhage may be present within the lesion.

Miscellaneous disorders

Carotid body tumor

Carotid body tumor (also known as chemodectoma, paraganglionoma) is a tumor of the glomus body (paraganglia). On angiography, there is characteristic splaying of the internal and carotid arteries (the 'inverted stirrup' sign) and a 'blush' by the tumor. CT demonstrates a markedly enhancing mass (see Fig. 24.25). On MR imaging there is, on T1 weighted sequences, a 'salt and pepper' appearance—the 'salt' representing hemorrhage,

and the 'pepper' signal, flow void. The condition may be sporadic or familial (autosomal dominant).

Laryngocele

A laryngocele is an acquired saccular swelling sited lateral to the thyrohyoid membrane and represents herniation of respiratory epithelium through a membrane defect. It can be identified on plain x-rays as an air shadow lateral to the larynx. CT will confirm the relationship to the thyrohyoid membrane.

Pharyngeal pouch

Pharyngeal pouch occurs between the two bands of the inferior constrictor muscle (Killian's dehiscence). The presentation is typically with the regurgitation of undigested food or occasionally with a neck lump in those over 50 years of age. Barium swallow appearances demonstrate filling of a pouch at the level of the lower cervical vertebrae (see Ch. 3).

Lipoma and sebaceous cyst

These two superficial lesions should be readily differentiated by ultrasound. A lipoma has echogenic characteristics which should be identical to the surrounding fatty tissues. A sebaceous cyst tends to be more hypoechoic and of a fluid nature. They also have characteristic appearances on MRI (see Fig. 24.26).

Fine needle aspiration cytology (FNAC) is the gold standard investigation for a neck mass.

Case conference

A 28-year-old lady was referred by her general practitioner with a right-sided neck mass. On examination, there was a firm swelling below and lateral to the right of the thyroid cartilage. No other abnormality was evident. She had no overt clinical features of thyroid disease.

Ultrasound of neck
A well-defined 1.8 × 2.3 cm hypoechoic mass is identified in the right lobe of

the thyroid. The mass is well encapsulated and predominantly solid, with some cystic spaces. Small areas of calcification are also noted. The remainder of the thyroid outlines normally. There is no significant lymphadenopathy. A subsequent isotope scan demonstrated a corresponding photopenic region within the right lobe. The appearances were felt to be consistent with a 'cold nodule.' Thyroid function tests were also normal.

Ultrasound-guided FNA
The procedure was explained, as were the risks, benefits and complications. Written and informed consent was obtained. Using an aseptic technique, a 21 gauge needle was advanced into the lesion under ultrasound control. Cells were aspirated, spread onto slides and sent to the cytology department.

A population of follicular cells was identified, and on this basis the patient was referred for thyroid surgery. The final histology was that of a follicular adenoma.

Conclusion
A hemithyroidectomy was performed. The patient's postoperative course was routine and she was discharged.

11. Neurological Symptoms

Neurological pathologies account for a significant proportion of hospital morbidity and mortality. Prompt medical and surgical management with appropriate imaging are crucial.

Unlike most other body systems, the plain film has only very limited application in neuroimaging. Its role is restricted to traumatic head injury and even then is of limited benefit. The mainstay of neuroimaging is computed tomography (CT), especially for trauma and suspected subarachnoid hemorrhage, and magnetic resonance imaging (MRI). The radiologist has an increasing role in the treatment of cerebral aneurysms by 'coiling' procedures.

Headache

Headache is a common complaint and is usually benign in nature. The vast majority of patients require no investigations; however, a detailed history is crucial as there are several 'red flags' (signs) that suggest potentially serious causes of headache.

Core symptoms prompting early radiological investigations
Sudden, severe headache

This is particularly relevant if found in association with nausea, vomiting, and neck stiffness. In this circumstance it is mandatory that subarachnoid hemorrhage (SAH) is excluded. Patients will often describe the headache as 'the worst of my life' and 'I thought I was going to die.' The investigation of choice is cranial CT.

SAH is confirmed by the presence of hyperdensity in the subarachnoid spaces (see Fig. 24.13). The patient requires additional imaging to visualize the intracranial vessels as, in 85% of such cases, the cause is a ruptured intracranial aneurysm. In 5% of cases, a ruptured arteriovenous malformation is the source and in 10% of patients no treatable cause is found. CT angiography (CTA) has replaced invasive catheter angiography in many centers (see Fig. 24.14), with catheter angiography reserved for inconclusive cases (see Fig. 24.7).

Headache worse in the mornings and/or on standing

Particularly in association with nausea and vomiting, this is suggestive of raised intracranial pressure (ICP) and is often due to the development of hydrocephalus. This is an increase in pressure within the ventricular system, due either to an obstruction of the cerebrospinal fluid (CSF) pathway or overproduction of CSF. Although initial investigation is usually CT, MRI is the investigation of choice. Obstruction to CSF flow can be produced by tumors or cysts, especially in the midline, involving the third or fourth ventricle.

On CT, the ventricles are seen to be dilated (see Fig. 24.18a), the earliest changes being seen in the temporal horns of the lateral ventricles.

A colloid cyst in the base of the septum pellucidum often obstructs the outflow from both lateral ventricles at the level of the foramina of Monroe (see Fig. 24.18). It can present with postural headaches and is a recognized cause of sudden death. On CT it is a low attenuation lesion seen at the foramen of Monroe. Signal characteristics are variable on MR depending on the protein content. There is no contrast enhancement on CT or MR.

In children, posterior fossa tumors are more common than supratentorial lesions and often present with hydrocephalus due to obstruction of the fourth ventricle (see Fig. 24.16). Excessive CSF production results in a non-obstructive (or communicating) hydrocephalus. Figure 24.15 demonstrates a lateral ventricular papilloma in a child, presenting with lethargy and sunset eyes. The latter is a classic finding in children with hydrocephalus.

Focal neurological deficit

Acute presentation

The presentation of a focal neurological deficit that is sudden and heralded as a unilateral limb weakness (hemiparesis) with or without speech difficulties (dysphasia) indicates a cerebrovascular accident (CVA) or stroke.

CT performed early after onset (less than 3 hours) is often normal, although early signs of infarction may be appreciated. Its primary role, however, is in detecting hemorrhagic transformation that would preclude antiplatelet or anticoagulant treatment. CT will also identify those patients with a large intracerebral hemorrhage (see Fig. 24.19). These present in a similar fashion but usually have significantly altered consciousness (decreased Glasgow Coma Scale) and/or a history of severe headache at onset.

Those hemorrhages centered on the basal ganglia and in the deep cerebellar hemisphere white matter are usually due to underlying hypertension. The hypertension produces arteriosclerotic changes in the perforator vessels supplying these territories, which results in a weakening within the vessel wall and a propensity to rupture. Other causes of intracerebral hemorrhage should also be considered.

Ruptured intracranial aneurysms can result in predominant intracerebral hematoma rather than subarachnoid hemorrhage (see Fig. 24.19). This classically occurs with middle cerebral artery aneurysms that rupture into the Sylvian fissure. Hemorrhage into pre-existing tumors may also occur.

Subacute presentation

A history of increasing neurological deficit over a period of time is more typical of a growing mass lesion, e.g., meningioma. The length of history reflects the nature of the underlying mass, with malignant tumors presenting within weeks, but more benign lesions over a period of months.

Cross-sectional imaging will identify and measure the dimensions of the mass. The location may be important in the differential diagnosis, e.g., sphenoidal ridge cerebellopontine angle (see Fig. 24.21). Characteristics of the mass may also provide further etiological clues: a mural nodule within the mass (cystic astrocytoma); calcification or dural tail (meningioma, see Fig. 24.20); cystic degeneration and necrosis (glioblastoma multiforme); or crossing the midline (butterfly glioma).

A group known generically as a 'white matter diseases' is the most common inflammatory disorder of the CNS. The most prevalent in the western world is multiple sclerosis, characterized by destruction of normally formed myelin, with relative axonal preservation. The etiology is unknown. Most patients present in the third or fourth decade. The first clinical symptom is often impaired or double vision (diplopia). Other common symptoms include weakness, tingling, numbness, and gait disturbances. With disease progression, loss of sphincter control, blindness, paralysis, and dementia may develop.

The diagnosis is fundamentally a clinical one; however, MRI sensitivity exceeds clinical examination alone as well as all other imaging modalities including CT. The diagnosis is usually made with reference to the clinical, laboratory, and imaging findings.

Multiple sclerosis is a clinical diagnosis supported by MRI findings.

MRI features include high signal on T2 weighted sequences in the periventricular white matter, often characteristically oval in shape ('Dawson's fingers'). These may be best appreciated in the sagittal images. Other common locations for demyelinating plaques are the corpus callosum and the craniocervical junction of the cord (classically C2 level; see Fig. 24.12).

Seizures

A seizure is the result of an abnormal electrical discharge within the brain. Epilepsy is a condition characterized by more than one seizure. The role of neuroimaging is to identify a structural epileptogenic focus. Symptomatic seizures may be acute due to a precipitant or remote to a pre-existent lesion, with seizure the main or only symptom. In adults acute symptomatic seizures are most commonly caused by trauma (see Fig. 24.10), cerebrovascular disease, tumors (see Fig. 24.3), drug withdrawal (including alcohol), CNS infection, and degenerative disease. In children with seizures, a metabolic disease should also be considered.

Remote seizures are caused by previous trauma, CVA, CNS infection, tumor, atrophy, malformations of cortical development, and hippocampal sclerosis (see Fig. 24.4).

Most of these causes are identifiable with CT or MRI, with the latter providing the better yield. For acute symptomatic seizure, CT is recommended. MRI should be arranged for non-acute symptomatic seizures with confusion and postictal deficit. In a child with unexplained cognitive or motor delays and less than 1 year of age, MRI is recommended. All patients with partial seizures, abnormal electroencephalograms (EEGs) and generalized epilepsy should also be imaged.

The nature of the seizure may indicate the location of a structural focus.

Head trauma

Traumatic brain injury (TBI) is a common cause of death and disability. The Center for Disease Control and Prevention (CDC) estimates that 2% of the US population, or 5.3 million Americans, have long term effects of TBI, needing help performing daily tasks. The annual incidence of head trauma is 1.4 million. Of these, 50,000 will die, 235,000 will be hospitalized, and another 1.1 million will be evaluated in an emergency department (ED). The leading causes of TBI are falls (28%), motor vehicle accidents (20%), being struck by or against an object (19%), and assaults (11%). Males are twice as likely as females to sustain TBI. Motor vehicle accidents are the major cause of TBI in the second and third decade. Falls account for most injuries in the elderly.

The principal imaging test in neurotrauma is CT, usually without contrast enhancement (non contrast CT). MRI has a limited role acutely. Clinical severity is assessed using the Glasgow Coma Scale (GCS). In mild head injury (GCS 13–15), observation is often all that is required. CT is reserved for those patients with persistent headache and/or vomiting. All patients with moderate (GCS 8–12) and severe (GCS less than 8) injury require imaging to detect hematomas requiring surgical intervention. The full extent of brain injury will not be completely determined with CT alone. Although MRI provides more accurate information regarding the prognosis,

limited availability in the acute setting limits its use.

Head injuries incurred can be classified into two groups:

- Primary lesions.
- Secondary lesions.

Primary lesions

Primary lesions are due to direct neuronal injury, primary hemorrhage and primary vascular injuries.

Primary neuronal

Nearly all primary neuronal injuries occur following shear-strain deformation by rotational acceleration of the head. Characteristic locations include diffuse axonal injuries (see Fig. 24.10b), cortical contusions, subcortical gray matter injury, and brain stem injury (see Fig. 24.10a). The sensitivity of CT in detecting these is low compared with MRI.

Primary hemorrhage

Primary hemorrhage results from injury to any of the cerebral vessels (meningeal, pial, artery, vein, capillary). The type of hemorrhage is dependent on the vessel injured.

Extradural hematoma

Extradural hematoma (EDH) is usually arterial and caused by direct laceration or tearing of meningeal arteries (often the middle meningeal artery) by skull fracture; these are often temporal or temporoparietal in location. Venous EDH is less common and results from laceration of a dural sinus by the fracture; these are usually in the posterior fossa.

On NCCT images, the EDH is identified as a biconvex ('lens shaped') area of high attenuation adjacent to the skull (see Fig. 24.11). An underlying fracture may be appreciated on the bony windows.

Subdural hematoma

Subdural hematoma (SDH) is typically caused by stretching and tearing of bridging veins that traverse the subdural space. The symptoms of an isolated SDH vary from asymptomatic to unconsciousness. The outcome is often poor due to secondary injuries and associated additional injuries.

On NCCT images, the SDH is identified as a crescentic mass adjacent to the skull bone (Fig. 11.1; see also Fig. 24.8). As a rule, acute SDH

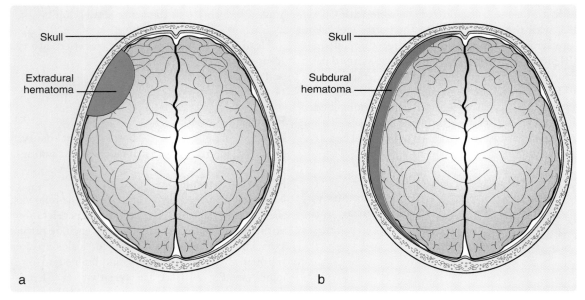

Fig. 11.1 Extradural (a) and subdural hematoma (b).

(within 2 weeks) is of higher attenuation than the brain, subacute SDH (2–4 weeks) isoattenuating with the brain, and chronic SDH (greater than 4 weeks) of lower attenuation than the brain.

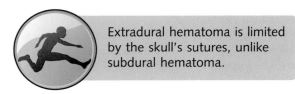

Extradural hematoma is limited by the skull's sutures, unlike subdural hematoma.

Intracerebral hematoma

Intracerebral hematoma (ICH) most commonly arises from rotational shear/strain injury to intraparenchymal arteries or veins. Occasionally direct penetrating injury to the vessel is the cause. Hematoma size varies from millimeters to several centimeters. ICH is usually within the frontal temporal white matter or basal ganglia.

On NCCT, these are high attenuation lesions with mass effect. If large, effacement of the ventricles and midline shift may be appreciated. It is important to look for 'contra-coup' injuries: with a frontal hematoma, review the occipital region for small petechial areas of high attenuation.

Intraventricular hemorrhage

Intraventricular hemorrhage (IVH) is quite common and can be caused by a variety of traumatic lesions, e.g., diffuse axonal injury (DAI), intracranial hemorrhage (ICH), and large contusions. It is most commonly due to tearing of subependymal veins within the ventricular walls. Traumatic SAH can also occur.

On NCCT there are high attenuation areas with fluid levels in the ventricles. The most common location is the occipital horns of the lateral ventricles.

Primary vascular

Primary vascular injuries include caroticocavernous fistulae (see Fig. 24.5), arterial dissections/occlusions, dural sinus lacerations and occlusions. There is often a significant delay from trauma to onset of symptoms. Those that are symptomatic are often unrecognized as they are masked by other intra- or extracranial injuries. Patients with basal skull fractures are particularly at risk (see Fig. 24.9).

Secondary effects of traumatic brain injury include arterial infarction, diffuse hypoxic injury (see Fig. 24.6), diffuse brain swelling/edema and pressure necrosis from brain displacement and herniation.

Case conference

A 42-year-old lady was admitted to the ED following collapse and loss of consciousness. Her husband, who had been at home with her, said that she had complained of a very severe headache for a short time prior to her collapse.

CT brain

On the unenhanced scan, there is hyperdensity in the subarachnoid spaces, most prominent in the right Sylvian fissure and the cisterna ambiens. There is no evidence of a mass lesion or midline shift. The appearances are consistent with subarachnoid hemorrhage.

A CT angiogram performed at the same time demonstrates a saccular enhancing lesion arising from the supraclinoid portion of the right internal carotid artery at the origin of the right posterior communicating (PCom) artery. The appearances are in keeping with a right PCom aneurysm.

After discussion with the neurosurgeons, it was agreed that endovascular occlusion was the preferred therapeutic option. The procedure was fully explained to the patient and her husband, together with the risks, benefits, and alternatives. Written and informed consent was obtained.

Endovascular occlusion

The patient underwent general anesthesia in the neurointerventional suite. A right femoral sheath was placed via Seldinger technique. Once full systemic heparinization was instituted, a guiding catheter was placed in the distal cervical right internal carotid artery. A coaxial catheter was advanced, through the guiding catheter, into the aneurysm sac at the level of the right PCom artery. Five detachable coils were deployed within the sac. The procedure was technically routine, with no complications recorded.

The patient was returned to the neurosurgical unit. Hydration was maintained (3 L in 24 hours). Close observations were instituted to check for evidence of stroke or hydrocephalus. The patient made a full neurological recovery.

Arrangements will be made for follow-up for a postcoiling catheter angiogram in 6 months to ensure that the sac remains occluded.

12. Urinary Tract Infection in Childhood

Children with a documented urinary tract infection (UTI) need to be investigated promptly and thoroughly, remembering the radiation dose that such examinations entail. The goals of imaging in UTI are to aid in the diagnosis of acute pyelonephritis, to identify those children who are at high risk of developing permanent renal damage, and to confirm and monitor the presence of renal scarring. Conditions that are associated with the development of long-term renal damage include obstructive uropathies (e.g., pelvi-ureteric junction obstruction), renal calculi, and congenital dysplastic kidneys.

UTIs are a common cause of morbidity in children. The term UTI, however, encompasses several different clinical conditions:

- Bacteriuria is defined as a colony count of $>10^5$/mL in a 'clean catch' (midstream, catheter, or suprapubic aspirate) specimen of urine.
- A lower UTI is diagnosed clinically when there is dysuria, frequency of micturition, and suprapubic tenderness in the absence of pyrexia.
- Acute pyelonephritis or an upper UTI is diagnosed when there is flank or abdominal pain, vomiting, and a pyrexia $> 38.5°C$, with cloudy or foul-smelling urine.
- The distinction between upper and lower urinary tract infections is clinically difficult but important, as permanent renal damage (scarring) may occur when the UTI involves the kidneys. There is an increased incidence of hypertension, complications during pregnancy, and renal failure in adulthood in those who develop renal scars as a child.

The current imaging guidelines as recommended by the American Academy of Pediatrics (AAP) are outlined in Figure 12.1. Local policies may vary somewhat.

Renal tract ultrasound

Ultrasound (US) defines the renal anatomy and will demonstrate any congenital abnormality such as a duplex or horseshoe kidney. Calculi are seen as echogenic (bright/white) foci. Scars may be seen as focal thinning of the renal cortex (more common in the upper and lower poles) or as a global reduction in the size of the kidney. Hydronephrosis is present when the renal pelvis and calyces are dilated, and the transverse diameter of the renal pelvis exceeds 1.0 cm. Neuropathic bladders are irregular in contour with thickened walls. Any sacculations and diverticula are seen as out-pouchings from the bladder wall.

Voiding cystourethrogram (VCUG)

A urinary catheter is inserted into the bladder and water-soluble contrast medium is then used to fill the bladder. Intermittent fluoroscopic images are obtained during bladder filling and micturition and demonstrate the outline of the bladder and the urethral contour (especially important in male infants). Vesico-ureteric reflux (VUR) is present when contrast flows retrogradely up the ureter(s) as the bladder is filled or during micturition (see Fig. 25.11). VUR is graded I–V depending on its severity.

DMSA Nuclear study

Tc^{99m} dimercaptosuccinic acid (DMSA) is administered intravenously. The dose depends on the child's weight. After 2 hours, images are obtained. The renal anatomy is demonstrated, as any functioning renal tissue will be outlined on the DMSA images. Renal scars manifest as defects in the renal outlines. The relative function of each kidney can be expressed as a percentage figure.

Other renal imaging investigations used in children with UTIs

VUR may also be detected directly by a nuclear cystogram, where pertechnetate is instilled directly into the bladder via a urinary catheter or indirectly when the child is imaged during micturition following an intravenous injection of Tc-labelled MAG-3.

AAP imaging guidelines for urinary tract infection in childhood

Age of patient	Imaging investigations*
<2 years	Renal US, VCUG, (+ DMSA if febrile)†
2–5 years	Renal US, VCUG†
>5 years	Renal US†

* Proven Proteus infection requires that an AXR be performed as *Proteus* sp. are associated with the formation of renal calculi.

† Voiding cystourethrogram (VCUG) is also performed if the renal ultrasound (US) shows a hydroureter or if the dimercaptosuccinic acid (DMSA) scan is abnormal.

Fig. 12.1 AAP imaging guidelines for urinary tract infection in childhood.

CT scans may be helpful when renal infection is thought to have spread beyond the capsule of the kidney or when the child has been infected with an unusual organism, such as *Candida* sp. or *Mycobacterium tuberculosis*. MRI is increasingly used in the detection of renal scarring.

The role of vesico-ureteric reflux

VUR occurs due to an inadequate length of the intravesical ureter. The natural history is for spontaneous cessation of VUR in the majority of children, vesico-ureteric junction competence developing with an increase in the length of the submucosal ureteric tunnel.

The relationship between acute pyelonephritis and VUR is not clear cut. VUR is reported to occur in 1–2% of healthy children and in almost two-thirds of children with UTIs. Importantly, there is an increased incidence of VUR in parents and siblings of children with reflux. VUR is also found in children with congenital and anatomical renal tract abnormalities. Such conditions include multicystic dysplastic kidney, pelvi-ureteric junction obstruction, and duplex renal systems. Finally, VUR is also found in children who have bladder outlet obstruction, and neuropathic or dysfunctional bladders.

Studies have shown that more severe VUR, in association with acute pyelonephritis, is more likely to result in the development of renal scars. However, not all children with VUR will develop renal damage, and some children with acute pyelonephritis who go on to develop renal scars do not have demonstrable VUR. To further complicate the issue, some children with VUR will develop renal scarring in the absence of UTI.

In other words, when there is VUR, both sterile and infected urine may be associated with the development of renal scars, but VUR is not a prerequisite for the development of renal damage in children with a history of acute pyelonephritis.

Case conference

A 4-month-old neonate was admitted last night with a 5-day history of vomiting and irritability. On examination he was dehydrated and his temperature was 39.5°C. He was tender to palpation in the left flank. His white cell count, ESR, and CRP were all elevated. His urine was cloudy and malodorous. It contained numerous pus cells. He was resuscitated with IV fluids and commenced on empirical antibiotic therapy. A suprapubic bladder tap was performed and the clean urine sample sent to microbiology for culture.

Renal tract ultrasound
The images show dilatation of the pelvi-calyceal systems and ureters bilaterally. On the right side there is a single collecting system. On the left side there is a duplex collecting system, with

complete duplication of the ureters to the level of the bladder. Both moieties of the duplex system are dilated. Posterior to the bladder all three dilated ureters can be seen. In addition, there is a soft tissue mass within the bladder, entered by one of the left-sided ureters. This is an ectopic ureterocele associated with the upper moiety of a duplex system. The collecting systems and ureters are filled with echogenic debris. This likely represents pyoureteronephrosis.

In a young male infant such as this, you also need to consider whether there is a bladder outlet obstruction, such as that caused by posterior urethral valves. Other than the ureterocele, the bladder appears normal on the ultrasound.

A voiding cystourethrogram (VCUG) should be performed to define the anatomy of the bladder and the urethra. The VCUG will also ascertain if the infant is refluxing into the dilated ureters.

Voiding cystourethrogram
The VCUG shows a filling defect on the left side of the bladder on the early filling views, consistent with the ureterocele seen on the ultrasound images. The bladder outline is otherwise normal and, when the infant voided, the urethra was seen to be normal in contour. During bladder filling, however, there was VUR into both the right renal tract and the lower moiety of the left renal tract at low volumes. The ureters are dilated bilaterally and the calyces are clubbed. This corresponds to grade IV VUR. There was no VUR into the upper moiety system of the left kidney, confirming that it is obstructed by the ureterocele.

- *Pediatric urologist*: I was asked to review this patient following his VCUG. His temperature has now settled on the antibiotic therapy. The urine cultures grew *Escherichia coli*. The patient is having a cystoscopy this afternoon, where we plan to incise the ureterocele to release the obstruction.
- *Pediatric radiologist*: This infant has had bilateral pyoureteronephrosis associated with a left-sided duplex system. He has bilateral dilating VUR. He is at increased risk for the development of renal scarring. I would suggest a DMSA scan in 6 months' time to look for this. If he has further urinary tract infections, then the first-line investigation will be a repeat ultrasound examination.

The vast majority of infants will pass meconium within the first 24 hours of life, and all should have done so by 48 hours of age. Delayed passage of meconium is normally associated with abdominal distension and vomiting (which may be bilious). In these circumstances, a supine abdominal radiograph and a contrast enema are indicated. The enema may be both diagnostic and therapeutic.

Figure 13.1 lists some of the more common causes of delayed passage of meconium in a newborn infant.

Think anatomically from the anal verge extending proximally. This will help you to remember both the anatomical and functional abnormalities that cause a neonatal low bowel obstruction.

Hirschsprung's disease

Hirschsprung's disease is a form of functional low bowel obstruction that is due to failure of caudal migration of neuroblasts in the developing bowel. The distal large bowel from the point of neuronal arrest to the anus is aganglionic. In about 75% of cases, the aganglionic segment extends only to the rectosigmoid region (short segment disease). Long segment disease involves a variable portion of the colon proximal to the sigmoid, and total aganglionosis coli the entire colon and a part of the terminal ileum. Approximately 5% of children with Hirschsprung's disease have Down's syndrome (see Fig. 25.5).

Severe bloody diarrhea, sepsis, and shock are associated with Hirschsprung's enterocolitis, which occurs in up to 30% of patients in both the pre- and postoperative period. Enterocolitis is the leading cause of death in Hirschsprung's disease and has an increased frequency in long segment disease. A suction or full thickness rectal biopsy is required for the definitive diagnosis of Hirschsprung's disease.

Meconium ileus

Meconium ileus is a form of distal intestinal obstruction caused by inspissated pellets of meconium in the terminal ileum. Over 90% of infants with meconium ileus have cystic fibrosis, and meconium ileus is the presenting feature of cystic fibrosis in 10–15% of affected patients. Of all patients with cystic fibrosis, those with the ΔF508 mutation (the most common) have a higher incidence of meconium ileus.

Over half of the affected infants have uncomplicated meconium ileus. In utero these babies produce meconium that is thick and tenacious, and that fills and distends the small bowel loops. The meconium desiccates in the terminal ileum and becomes impacted, causing a high grade obstruction. A functional microcolon results. Meconium ileus is described as complicated when intra-uterine volvulus, atresia, gangrene, perforation, or meconium peritonitis supervenes.

Functional immaturity of the colon

Immature left colon (also known as meconium plug syndrome or small left colon) is a relatively common cause of neonatal bowel obstruction.

Risk factors include premature infants, those born by cesarean section, maternal diabetes and drug ingestion, and infants whose mothers were treated with magnesium sulfate (for pre-eclampsia) during labor. The condition is *not* associated with cystic fibrosis. The exact cause of the syndrome remains unknown, but immaturity of the myenteric plexus had been postulated as a theory.

Ileal atresia

Jejunal and ileal atresias have a common etiology and are due to an intrauterine vascular accident. As with the duodenum, atresia is more common than stenosis, and the proximal jejunum and distal ileum are more frequently affected.

Delayed passage of meconium
• Hirschsprung's disease
• Meconium ileus
• Functional immaturity of the colon
• Ileal or colonic atresia
• Anorectal malformations
• Small bowel malrotation and volvulus
• Omphalomesenteric duct remnants
• Extrinsic compression of the distal bowel by a mass lesion
• Paralytic ileus, sepsis, drugs and metabolic upset

Fig. 13.1 Delayed passage of meconium.

VACTERL*	
V	Vertebral segmentation anomalies
A	Anorectal malformation
C	Congenital heart disease
T	Tracheo-esophageal fistula
E	Esophageal atresia
R	Renal anomalies
L	Limb anomalies (typically radial ray defects)

* Two or more components of the VACTERL sequence of malformations must be present for the infant to be labelled as belonging to this group.

Fig. 13.2 VACTERL.

Anorectal malformations

The incidence of anorectal malformations (also known as imperforate anus or anorectal atresia) varies between 1 in 1500 and 1 in 5000 live births. The precise etiology is unknown, but the condition results from failure of descent and separation of the hindgut and the genito-urinary tract during the second trimester. The abnormality consists of anorectal atresia, with or without an anomalous connection between the atretic anorectum and the genito-urinary tract.

Associated congenital anomalies are common. The VACTERL sequence occurs in around 45% of patients (Fig. 13.2).

Anorectal atresias are classified into high or low lesions, depending upon whether the rectum ends above or below the puborectalis sling. The distinction between high and low lesions is clinical rather than radiological, and has important therapeutic and prognostic consequences.

In both males and females with low lesions, there is usually a visible perineal opening. The orifice may be located more anteriorly than normal (an ectopic anus) and it may be stenotic or covered with a membrane. Low lesions do not have a communication with the genito-urinary tract. Females with low lesions will have separate urethral and vaginal orifices with an intact hymen. Low lesions also include isolated rectal atresia or stenosis. This type of lesion is treated surgically with an anoplasty or dilatation soon after birth.

In both males and females with high lesions, no visible perineal fistula is present. Male patients will usually have a fistulous tract between the atretic anorectum and the posterior urethra. Less commonly there is a fistula to the bladder or anterior urethra. Female patients have fistulae from the atretic anorectum to the vagina or vestibule. Rarely, in both male and female patients, the rectum ends blindly. High lesions are initially managed with a colostomy to divert the fecal stream away from the genito-urinary tract. Definitive repair is performed at a later stage.

Colonic atresia

Colon atresia is rare when compared with other intestinal atresias, and colonic stenosis is rarer still. The right colon is most commonly affected.

It is thought to be due to an in utero vascular accident.

Radiological investigations

Abdominal x-ray (AXR)

This will show multiple, dilated loops of bowel down to the level of the obstruction, without distal gas. This appearance is referred to as a neonatal 'low bowel obstruction,' i.e., the obstruction lies distal to the mid-ileum. In addition, there may or may not be a mottled fecal pattern seen in the right iliac fossa (the 'soap bubble' pattern; classically said to be diagnostic of meconium ileus, but is also seen with other causes of distal ileal obstruction).

Differentiation between small and large bowel on the AXR to determine the precise level of the obstruction is virtually impossible in the neonate. Both small and large bowel may be of similar caliber proximal to an obstruction, and the haustra are poorly developed in the neonatal bowel.

A neonatal 'high bowel obstruction' is present when the obstruction lies proximal to the mid-ileum. The AXR will show only a few dilated loops of bowel. Regardless of the cause, all neonates with a high bowel obstruction need urgent surgical referral, rather than further radiological investigation.

Contrast enema

It is important to ensure that the infant is fully resuscitated prior to the examination, and that IV fluids continue to run during the procedure. Water-soluble contrast medium is used, all types of which are hypertonic to the infant's plasma, placing the baby at risk of dehydration due to osmolar fluid shifts.

A supine view of the abdomen is initially required to exclude a complicating perforation. With the infant in the left lateral position, the tip of a Foley catheter is inserted just inside the anal margin. A small amount of contrast is hand injected. At this stage of the examination the radiologist is looking to exclude rectosigmoid Hirschsprung's disease. The following signs are present on the enema in this condition:

- There is a funnel-shaped zone of transition between the more proximal dilated (ganglionated) bowel and the distal narrow (denervated) bowel.
- The rectosigmoid ratio is reversed (i.e., the sigmoid colon has a greater diameter than the

rectum; normally, the rectum is the most distensible part of the bowel).
- Abnormal muscle contractions may be observed in the denervated distal bowel.

The catheter balloon must never be inflated early on during the enema. At best the transition zone in Hirschsprung's disease would be missed and, at worst, a stiff, aganglionic rectum would be perforated.

If a low, rectosigmoid Hirschsprung's disease is excluded, the catheter may be inserted further and its balloon gently inflated, to act as a seal and prevent contrast leakage. The baby is placed supine and further contrast is injected. In all other causes of a low obstruction, the colon distal to the point of obstruction will be reduced in caliber. This is known as a *microcolon* and is due to colonic disuse in utero. The aim of the enema is to discover the precise level of the obstruction and, if possible, to run the contrast into the dilated, meconium-laden loops of bowel proximal to the point of obstruction. The enema then becomes both therapeutic and diagnostic. Water is drawn into the bowel lumen by osmosis, mixes with the tenacious meconium, loosens it and allows it to pass.

Infants with meconium ileus and functional immaturity of the colon will generally pass large quantities of meconium immediately following a successful enema, and their obstruction is relieved. Failure to relieve the bowel obstruction in meconium ileus may necessitate a second enema in the following days. Should this also fail to relieve the infant's symptoms, then surgery would usually be required. All infants with bowel atresias, stenoses, webs, and Hirschsprung's disease need surgical intervention.

In an infant with functional immaturity of the colon, there is generally an abrupt change in colonic caliber seen at the level of the splenic flexure. It can be difficult to distinguish this condition from long segment Hirschsprung's disease with a transition zone at this level, and biopsy may later be required to confirm the presence of ganglion cells in the descending colon.

Case conference

The surgical team were asked to review a 2-day-old term neonate in the nursery by the pediatricians. The history was of progressive abdominal distension, failure to pass meconium, and onset of bilious vomiting.

Abdominal radiographs
The supine abdominal x-ray demonstrates several distended loops of bowel throughout the abdomen. There is no gas seen in the rectum. It is impossible in a neonate to tell whether the distended loops are small or large bowel, as the valvulae conniventes and haustral pattern have not yet developed. However, given the number of dilated loops, the picture is that of a low bowel obstruction, i.e., the obstruction lies between the distal ileum and the anorectum. Low bowel obstructions in neonates should be investigated with a contrast enema. The enema is useful to determine the cause of the obstruction, be it mechanical or functional. In certain circumstances it may also be therapeutic.

(Neonatal contrast enemas are performed using a water-soluble contrast medium that is hypertonic to the infant's plasma. In cases of mechanical obstruction due to inspissated meconium, such as meconium ileus, the hypertonic fluid will draw extracellular water into the bowel lumen by osmosis and loosen off the meconium plugging the bowel lumen. In successful enemas, the infant will then pass this meconium and the obstruction will be relieved.)

Contrast enema
The enema images show an extremely narrow caliber colon. This is a microcolon—the colon of disuse. Contrast was run proximally to the cecum and refluxed through the ileocecal valve into the terminal ileum. The ileum outlined by the contrast is also reduced in caliber. Only a few centimeters of small bowel are delineated and the contrast did not reach the dilated bowel loops. The implication is that the obstruction is mechanical and in the distal ileum. In meconium ileus we would expect to see filling defects in the bowel lumen of the terminal ileum due to the meconium pellets and to be able to run the contrast into the dilated bowel loops proximal to the luminal obstruction. This is not true of this case and therefore the radiological diagnosis is one of distal ileal atresia.

- *Pediatric surgeon*: This is generally an isolated congenital abnormality due to an ischemic bowel injury. This may be a primary vascular accident or possibly secondary to an in utero mechanical obstruction such as a volvulus. The baby is scheduled for a laparotomy this afternoon.

14. A Limp in Childhood

Children not infrequently present with an inability to weight bear or a limp. The limp may be secondary to pain, or a structural hip or lower limb deformity. Clinically, it is important to try to localize any pain the child may have. Associated symptoms (such as fever) should be recorded and the time course of the symptoms noted. Radiologically, the most common causes of a limp tend to be classified according to anatomic regions and the age of the patient. Some of the more common causes of a limp are outlined in Figure 14.1 and discussed in brief.

Developmental dysplasia of the hip (DDH)

The term developmental dysplasia of the hip (DDH) refers to an abnormal relationship between the femoral head and the acetabulum. Most cases of DDH are thought to be due to ligamentous laxity and a high level of maternal estrogens. Risk factors include a positive family history, an abnormal position in utero, being of Caucasian racial origin or being papoosed with the hips in adduction, such as is traditional with Native American infants. Girls are much more commonly affected than boys. DDH is bilateral in up to one-third of cases. DDH may be clinically suspected if there are asymmetric gluteal folds, foot deformities, or a positive Ortolani or Barlow test. Infants are usually screened if there is a positive family history or if they have been born by breech delivery.

Ultrasound of the hips is the imaging method of choice in young infants (see Fig. 25.6). In those children who have ossified femoral heads, an anteroposterior (AP) radiograph of the pelvis is performed. This is the first investigation used in those children who present late. The acetabular roof is steep and the femoral head is displaced superolaterally in infants with dysplastic hip joints. In addition, the ossification center for the femoral head is small on the affected side.

Non-ionizing radiation techniques should be maximized in children.

Transient synovitis of the hip

Transient synovitis (irritable hip) is a common, non-traumatic cause of a limp in the younger child. The cause is unknown and the onset of symptoms acute. A hip joint effusion is present in the majority of patients. The diagnosis is one of exclusion, the differential diagnoses including septic arthritis, inflammatory arthritides, leukemia, and trauma. Ultrasound of the hip joints and plain radiographs are the initial imaging investigations. The latter will be normal in this group of patients. The joint fluid, if aspirated, is sterile in patients with transient synovitis. Management is by bed rest, together with analgesics if required.

Septic arthritis

Septic arthritis refers to a joint infection and is usually due to pyogenic organisms. In infants and young children, infection spreads from the metaphysis, via the epiphyseal plate, to the epiphysis and joint space. In older children, spread is from an adjacent focus of osteomyelitis.

Ultrasound and plain radiographs of the hips are taken initially. Ultrasound can also be used to guide aspiration of fluid from the joint, which can then be sent for microbacterial analysis. The plain films may be normal early in the course of the illness. Destruction of the epiphysis and dislocation of the hip may be seen later on and in complicated cases. Skeletal scintigraphy is useful to exclude an associated osteomyelitis, and would show increased uptake on all phases of a three-phase examination.

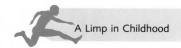

Common causes of a limp	
Age of patient	Causes of a limp
Up to 3 years	Developmental dysplasia of the hip, transient synovitis, septic arthritis, discitis, neuromuscular disorders
3–10 years	Perthes' disease, discitis (especially preschool children), inflammatory arthritides, Blount's disease
Adolescents	Slipped capital femoral epiphysis, discitis
Any age	Trauma, osteomyelitis, leg length discrepancy, bone tumors

Fig. 14.1 Common causes of a limp.

Septic arthritis requires urgent treatment to prevent joint destruction.

Perthes' disease

Perthes' disease (Legg–Calvé–Perthes' disease) is idiopathic avascular necrosis of the immature capital femoral epiphysis. The condition most commonly presents between the ages of 4 and 10 years, with boys being more often affected. Clinically, the child presents with hip or knee pain and a limp. The condition is bilateral in approximately 10% of cases.

Early changes in the bone include subchondral fissure fractures, and sclerosis and irregularity of the epiphysis. Later, the femoral head fragments and collapses. The femoral neck may broaden and develop cystic change. Repair and re-ossification occur gradually, along with remodeling. The final contour of the bony epiphysis depends upon the original extent of the avascular necrosis and the patient's management. Initially, the patient is imaged using plain radiographs of the hips (see Fig. 25.14). MRI and isotope bone scans are helpful in the early stages if the plain films are normal. Bone marrow edema can be demonstrated with MRI, and lack of femoral head enhancement following IV gadolinium (contrast) supports the diagnosis of avascular necrosis. At scintigraphy, lack of tracer uptake by the femoral head is seen with avascular necrosis.

Treatment is aimed at keeping the femoral head contained by the acetabulum, protecting the articular cartilage and reducing the stress on the femoral head as it re-ossifies. Degenerative disease of the hip joint is a common late sequela.

Perthes' disease more commonly presents between the ages of 4 and 8 years; slipped capital femoral epiphysis (SCFE) occurs in adolescents.

Slipped capital femoral epiphysis (SCFE)

Slipped capital (or upper) femoral epiphysis (SCFE) is a hip disorder of adolescence. Most cases are regarded as idiopathic, although it is thought that it may be a hormone-mediated process, given its occurrence around the time of the pubertal growth spurt. In up to one-third of patients, SCFE is a bilateral, though asymmetric, condition.

The lesion of SCFE is analogous to a Salter I fracture across the proximal femoral growth plate. The femoral head slips posteriorly and medially. The abnormal position of the femoral head is best seen on the frog-leg lateral radiograph. The AP radiograph may be normal, or there may be subtle broadening of the growth plate and a reduced height of the femoral head (see Fig. 25.15). Further slippage is prevented by pinning of the femoral head in place (it is *not* manipulated back to the anatomical position). Chondrolysis of the articular cartilage of the femoral head and avascular necrosis are the two most significant complications and may occur pre- and post-pinning.

Toddler's fracture

Toddler's fracture is the synonym used to describe an undisplaced spiral or oblique tibial fracture that occurs in children between the ages of 9 months to 3 years when they are beginning to weightbear. These children present with a history of a limp or refusal to bear weight. A history of trauma may not be elicited. The initial radiographs are often normal. The children are usually treated symptomatically in a cast. Repeat x-rays after 10–14 days will confirm a healing fracture.

Discitis

Infection involving the intervertebral disc and/or the adjacent vertebral body endplates leads to severe back pain and muscle spasm. Limping is more common in younger children. The infection is usually low grade, with *Staphylococcus* as the underlying organism. Systemic signs tend to be minimal. Diagnosis is often difficult, as plain radiographs may be normal for several weeks. MRI is the most helpful imaging technique as it will confirm disc space narrowing and edema of the adjacent vertebral bodies. Intravenous gadolinium is helpful in detecting complications such as a paravertebral or extradural abscess. Patients with discitis are treated with antibiotics, analgesics, and bed rest.

Radiological evaluation

Pelvic radiographs

Two views of the pelvis are usually performed in children and adolescents. These are the straight AP view and the 'frog leg' lateral (Lowenstein) view. The knees are bent up and the hips are then abducted. Plain radiographs of the hips are taken in all children who present with a limp, unless there is a definite predisposing factor (e.g., trauma) or focal signs directing the clinician elsewhere, on clinical examination.

Radiographs of the lumbar spine

Lower back pain is a relatively common complaint in children and adolescents, usually due to soft tissue injury. Persistent back pain in this age group, however, is a symptom that must be taken seriously. Plain radiographs of the lumbar spine are the first-line imaging investigation, but it should be remembered that they are a high radiation dose examination. Radiographs are useful in the setting of trauma and also when looking for signs of inflammation (osteomyelitis and discitis), benign and malignant spinal tumors, and congenital spinal abnormalities (including scoliosis).

In the setting of persistent lower back pain with normal radiographs, the child should proceed to an isotope bone scan and/or an MRI of the lumbar spine.

Ultrasound scan of the hips

The best way of detecting a hip joint effusion is by ultrasound. Each hip is scanned in turn using a high frequency linear probe. The joint capsule is seen as an echogenic line, which normally runs parallel to the femoral neck. When a joint effusion is present, the joint capsule has a convex anterior margin, and the joint space is widened by the anechoic fluid. The depth of the effusion may be measured between the femoral neck and the joint capsule. A value greater than 4 mm or a difference between the two sides of greater than 2 mm is considered significant.

Ultrasound of the hips to look for dysplasia

This examination can only be performed in young infants before the femoral head has ossified (usually around 4–6 months of age). Each hip is scanned in turn using a high frequency linear probe. The ultrasound probe is held longitudinally over the hip joint. The iliac bone is seen in profile, along with the acetabular roof, triradiate cartilage, cartilaginous labrum and the unossified femoral head. The femoral head should be one-half to two-thirds covered by the acetabular roof, and the iliac bone and acetabulum should form a sharp angle together.

Isotope bone scans (scintigraphy)

Methylene diphosphonate (MDP) is labelled with Tc^{99m} and injected into the patient (see Part II, Principles of Radiology). The dose of the radiopharmaceutical administered is dependent upon the child's weight. The isotope is taken up in areas of active bone metabolism. The examination may be performed as either a three-phase or a static scan. In the former, images are obtained in the vascular (immediate), blood pool (after about 5 minutes), and static (after about 2 hours) phases. This type of scan is useful to investigate suspected inflammatory bone disease, infection, or trauma.

A static scan alone is useful in the detection of both benign and malignant bone tumors, and also has a place in the investigation of children with lower back pain, osteomyelitis, and Perthes' disease. When there is avascular necrosis, no isotope is taken up (a 'cold spot'). Magnification of the relevant areas with a pinhole collimator is a useful technique in pediatric patients, particularly in the assessment of lesions adjacent to the metabolically active epiphyseal plate. Tomographic scintigraphy (SPECT) is particularly helpful in the evaluation of spinal abnormalities.

Isotope bone scans should always be interpreted alongside plain radiographs of the area under investigation.

CT scan of the hips

This is rarely done outside the setting of trauma. However, it is increasingly used in infants and older children with DDH who have had failed conservative management.

Infants with DDH occasionally have CT scans performed to confirm the correct position of the femoral heads relative to the acetabula, once they are in spica casts (plaster casts that hold the hips in abduction).

MRI of the hips and pelvis

Use of MRI tends to be reserved for those children in whom a diagnosis cannot be made by a combination of ultrasound, plain radiographs, and scintigraphy, or those children with complications of their primary pathology. MRI has the advantage of not using ionizing radiation, but has the disadvantage of requiring sedation or anesthesia in younger children. It is particularly useful in examining the cartilaginous structures of the hip, such as the labrum in DDH. It is also useful, acutely, in children with suspected bone and joint infection or avascular necrosis of the femoral head.

Case conference

A 9-year-old boy originally presented with a 3-day history of severe left-sided hip pain and a limp. On examination, the left leg was held adducted and externally rotated. Passive abduction, flexion and internal rotation were all decreased. The child's past history revealed that he had complained of an ache in his left groin over the past 2 months. He was on regular peritoneal dialysis, having been born with posterior urethral valves and subsequently developing renal failure.

AP and Lowenstein views of both hips were obtained. These show an abnormal bone texture, with mixed areas of sclerosis and reduced bone density. There is widening of the proximal femoral growth plate on the right side and irregularity of the symphysis pubis. These features are consistent with renal osteodystrophy. On the left side, the femoral head has slipped posteriorly and medially. This is seen best on the Lowenstein view. The diagnosis is left-sided slipped capital (upper) femoral epiphysis, secondary to renal osteodystrophy.

The patient was taken to OR and the epiphysis was pinned in place. That was 2 months ago. The patient has now re-presented with increasing pain in both hips.

- *Pediatric radiologist*: The new AP and Lowenstein views of the pelvis again show the bone changes of renal osteodystrophy. Two screws are seen along the left femoral neck, passing into the left femoral head. Note that the position of the left femoral head has not changed since the initial films, the pins having prevented further slippage of the epiphysis. However, the procedure has been complicated by the development of avascular necrosis (AVN) in the left capital femoral epiphysis. The height of the epiphysis is reduced, its outline is irregular and it is very sclerotic. On the right side, the capital femoral epiphysis has also started to slip; it has moved posteriorly and medially.

- *Orthopedic surgeon*: The new slip of the right capital femoral epiphysis requires pinning. In addition, given the development of AVN in the left femoral head, the pins on the left side need to be removed or retracted to prevent the development of chondrolysis (articular cartilage necrosis of the femoral head).
- *Pediatric radiologist*: Given that he has renal osteodystrophy, he is at risk of epiphyseal slippage at other sites, particularly at the wrist. This should be borne in mind if he complains of pain in other joints.

15. Pregnancy

Obstetric ultrasound is used both for routine assessment to confirm pregnancy has occurred and that its milestones have been achieved. In addition, fetal and maternal abnormalities are assiduously checked for.

First trimester ultrasound

This is intended to fulfil the following functions:
- Confirmation of pregnancy.
- Confirmation of dates.
- Threatened abortion.
- Suspected multiple gestation.
- Suspected ectopic pregnancy.
- Screening for fetal abnormality.
- Molar pregnancy.

Confirmation of pregnancy
Ultrasound is used to determine the presence of the gestation sac, yolk sac, fetal pole (embryo), amnion, and cardiac activity. The gestational sac is not visible until it is 2–3 mm in size (at 4.5 weeks) and it increases by 1 mm per day.

Transvaginal ultrasound scanning (TVUS) will demonstrate structures and confirm viability about 1 week earlier than transabdominal scanning (TAS).

TAS is performed initially but if its findings are inconclusive or too early to confirm viability, then TVUS is used. A full maternal bladder is essential for TAS in early pregnancy but must be empty for TVUS. The fetal pole should be reliably seen by weeks 5–6 on TVUS and by week 7 on TAS. Fetal cardiac activity should now be visible and a viable pregnancy can be confidently diagnosed.

Confirmation of dates
Clinical dating of a pregnancy is based on the patient's recollection of the first day of her last menstrual period (LMP) and on the estimation of uterine size. Both these methods are prone to inaccuracy.

Ultrasound milestones in the first trimester are a much more accurate means of assessing gestational age from 5 weeks onwards. The earliest accurate method is by measuring the gestational sac diameter, circumference or volume at 5–6 weeks.

After 6 weeks the fetal pole is reliably visualized and a crown–rump length (CRL) measurement is performed. CRL is the maximum length of the fetal pole from the top of the head to rump excluding limb buds and yolk sac. CRL measurement is accurate from 6–12 weeks (±5 days).

Threatened abortion
Threatened abortion is the association of vaginal bleeding and cramping within the first 20 weeks of pregnancy. The possible findings on ultrasound include:
- *Viable pregnancy*: A gestation sac with a viable fetal pole correctly implanted in the uterine cavity.
- *Incomplete abortion*: Some of the products of conception may have passed but the uterus may contain an ill-defined sac or mass. No viable fetus.
- *Complete abortion*: An enlarged uterus in keeping with early pregnancy but no evidence of sac or fetal pole. Thickened decidual reaction may be visible in the endometrium.
- *Missed abortion*: The gestation sac and fetal pole are visible but there is no evidence of viability (a fetal pole larger than 5 mm should show cardiac activity).
- *Anembryonic pregnancy*: Blighted ovum, in which the sac develops but the fetus does not. Ultrasound demonstrates an empty sac, usually larger than expected for dates. A mean sac diameter greater than 2.5 cm and no fetal pole is diagnostic of a blighted ovum (TAS). A small empty sac could be due to incorrect dates. If the diagnosis is in doubt, either use TVUS or rescan TAS in 7–10 days.

Suspected multiple gestation

Check for the presence of more than one gestational sac (dizygotic/fraternal) or more than one fetal pole in a single sac (monozygotic/identical). Multiple pregnancies have an incidence of 1%, of which approximately two-thirds are dizygotic/polyzygotic.

In early first trimester, bleeding at the site of implantation may mimic a second sac—two fetal poles should be identified before making the diagnosis of multiple pregnancy. It is important to determine chorionicity in early pregnancy due to the higher incidence of fetal abnormalities and complications in monochorionic pregnancy.

Between 6 and 9 weeks, dichorionic twins have a thick separating membrane > 2 mm in diameter. After 9 weeks the membrane becomes progressively thinner and measurement less reliable. In dichorionic twins the junction of the membrane with the sac wall gives a characteristic 'lambda' sign.

 When one sac is identified, search for two. When two sacs are identified, search for three, and so on ...

Suspected ectopic pregnancy

The patient will present with a positive pregnancy test, pelvic pain, abnormal vaginal bleeding, and will possibly be in shock. There may be a clinical suspicion of a pelvic mass. If ultrasound shows an intrauterine pregnancy, then a coexistent ectopic is highly unlikely (incidence of 1 in 30,000). Possible US findings are of a complex adnexal mass with fluid in the pouch of Douglas (blood) and a fluid collection in the endometrium (pseudosac).

TVUS may show an extrauterine sac with a live embryo. This is conclusive of an ectopic pregnancy but only represents 5% of cases.

Screening for fetal abnormality

Ultrasound can be used to measure the nuchal translucency (NT) at the back of the fetal neck. An NT > 3 mm increases the fetal risk for chromosomal abnormalities, especially trisomy 21 (Down's syndrome). NT is usually used in conjunction with maternal age and biochemical triple screening to assess an individual's risk.

Counselling on the risk value is an integral part of the test.

Ultrasound may also demonstrate some gross fetal abnormalities, such as anencephaly, towards the end of the first trimester.

Molar pregnancy (gestational trophoblastic disease)

The patient may present with painless vaginal bleeding, excessive vomiting and high blood pressure.

US will show a uterus filled with an endometrial mass with or without cystic spaces ('snowstorm' appearance). In 50% of cases large cysts containing septa may be present in the ovaries (theca luteal cysts). These are thought to be due to increased levels of circulating human chorionic gonadotrophin (HCG). Occasionally an anembryonic sac may be seen.

Molar pregnancy can be partial or complete. Partial moles may have a coexistent fetus or fetal parts but these are not present in a complete molar pregnancy. Although benign, molar pregnancies may predispose to an invasive mole or the development of choriocarcinoma.

Second trimester ultrasound

Indications include:
- Assess fetal normality.
- Confirmation of dates.
- Adjunct to amniocentesis.
- Raised maternal serum alphafetoprotein.

Assess fetal normality

US is an essential tool in detecting major and minor fetal structural abnormalities and requires a skilled and experienced operator. It will not detect all fetal abnormalities. It must be performed before 24 weeks if termination of pregnancy is an option. It is commonly offered to all pregnant mothers as part of a screening test in association with maternal serum alphafetoprotein levels (MSAFP) levels. Anomalies detectable by US are as follows.

Neural tube defects (NTDs)

Incidence of 5 per 1000 births; predominantly anencephaly and spina bifida (SB) (95%).

Anencephaly

Absence of cranial vault and cerebral hemispheres. Evident on view for biparietal diameter (BPD) and sagittal section. Fetus still moves and kicks. May have associated spinal lesions (50%). Can be diagnosed after 11 weeks.

Encephalocele
Five percent of NTDs. Defect in cranium usually occipital (75%) with associated herniated fluid-filled or brain-filled cysts.

Spina bifida
Usually detected by recognizing associated defects in the skull, which act as markers: frontal bone scalloping ('lemon' sign) and/or anterior elongated curvature of the cerebellum ('banana' sign). Spina bifida is visible as widening of the fetal spine with a posterior cyst, filled with either fluid or spinal cord. Ventriculomegaly is usually present.

Cranial disorders
Ventriculomegaly
Increase in size of ventricles, usually lateral. Early enlargement is diagnosed by measuring the diameter at the level of the atrium (abnormal > 10 mm). Incidence of 2 per 1000 births. It is usually caused by obstruction which may be internal or external.

Dandy–Walker syndrome
Visible on US as a large posterior fossa cyst (dilated fourth ventricle). The cerebellum may be splayed with the vermis absent. Incidence of 1 per 30,000 births.

Agenesis of the corpus callosum (CC)
The CC is composed of nerve fibers connecting two cerebral hemispheres at the cavum septum pellucidum (CSP). Absence of CSP at BPD level may indicate diagnosis.

Holoprosencephaly
The brain fails to divide into two halves, resulting in little or no visible midline echo (falx). A single dilated lateral ventricle is visible. There are three main types depending on the degree of cleavage: lobar, semi-lobar, and alobar.

Microcephaly
Small brain, small head. Diagnosed by serial measurements of head to abdomen circumference ratios.

Cardiac conditions potentially detectable using ultrasound
• Dextrocardia
• Atrial and ventricular septal defects
• Univentricular heart
• Hypoplastic left ventricle
• Pulmonary stenosis and atresia
• Transposition of the great vessels
• Tetralogy of Fallot
• Ebstein's anomaly
• Double outlet ventricle
• Dysrhythmias—ectopics, supraventricular tachycardia, complete heart block

Fig. 15.1 Cardiac conditions potentially detectable using ultrasound.

Cardiac disorders
This is the largest group of congenital abnormalities and accounts for 1% of all abnormalities at birth. They range in severity and may be isolated or associated with other conditions. Diagnosis depends on the demonstration of the four chambers and right and left outflow tracts on a transverse section of the fetal heart. It is important to recognize the foramen ovale as a normal defect between the atria and that the normal fetal heart rate is 120–160 bpm.

The conditions outlined in Figure 15.1 are potentially detectable using US.

Thoracic disorders
Congenital cystic adenomatoid malformation (CCAM)
A condition of the fetal lung involving the development of cysts of various sizes. Usually unilateral (85%).

Lung sequestration
A bright mass usually located in the lower lobes of the lung may correspond to a sequestrated lobe. This lobe has a separate blood supply and has no connection to the airways.

Pleural effusion
Appearance of fluid at the base of the fetal lungs—may be either unilateral or bilateral

('batwing' appearance). May be associated with other conditions such as hydrops fetalis.

Diaphragmatic hernia
Incidence of 1 per 4000 births. Although the diaphragm is difficult to image, the associated pathology will lead to the diagnosis. Check for the position of the fetal stomach: if a cystic mass is present in the thorax and no stomach is seen in the left upper abdomen then a left-sided hernia is present. The heart is also displaced to the right. Left-sided hernia is more common than right-sided.

Abdominal disorders
These may be divided into three main groups: abdominal wall, gastrointestinal tract, and urinary tract.

Abdominal wall defects
Omphalocele   This is characterized by a sac anterior to the abdominal wall, covered by a layer of peritoneum. The sac contains solid and cystic components representing the liver, stomach, and bowel. It is a midline defect and the umbilical cord enters at the apex of the sac. Check for other fetal abnormalities.

Gastroschisis   An isolated condition in which a defect is present, usually to the right of the cord insertion. Fetal bowel can be seen freely floating in the amniotic fluid. There is no covering membrane.

Gastrointestinal disorders
Abnormalities of the gastrointestinal system usually result in increased amniotic fluid levels (polyhydramnios) due to impaired fetal swallowing.

Esophageal atresia   In 10% of cases complete atresia results in no stomach being visible on US, and associated polyhydramnios. The majority of cases have an associated tracheo-esophageal fistula, which may cause the stomach to fill and make antenatal diagnosis difficult.

Duodenal and jejunal atresia   A double or triple bubble appearance in the upper abdomen, caused by a dilated proximal gastrointestinal tract.

Abdominal cysts   Fluid-filled cysts may be identified in the fetal abdomen arising from the liver, biliary tree (choledochal cysts), ovary, or mesentery.

Urinary tract disorders
Obstructive lesions are associated with reduced amniotic fluid (oligohydramnios). Normal US must show both kidneys and a fluid-filled bladder. Abnormalities range from simple cysts to lethal conditions.

Renal agenesis   Bilateral agenesis is lethal. Failure to show the fetal bladder (no urine production) or either kidney with no amniotic fluid is consistent with the diagnosis. Incidence of 1 per 5000 births. May be unilateral (1 per 2000 births). Affected babies have a normal prognosis.

Infantile polycystic kidney disease   Always bilateral. Appear as large echobright kidneys due to microcystic appearance.

Obstructive uropathies   This describes a large range of conditions and US appearances. There may be mild unilateral renal dilatation to severe bilateral hydronephrosis caused by urethral stenosis. US will demonstrate fluid in the renal collecting systems with reduced levels of renal cortical tissue and decreased amniotic fluid.

Skeletal disorders
Ultrasound can demonstrate conditions that cause limb shortening or absence of all or part of a limb.

Confirmation of dates
Fetal biometry can be performed during the second trimester to confirm the menstrual dates and set a delivery date. Confirmation of dates is also essential for any follow-up growth scans. The routine measurements performed are as follows.

Biparietal diameter
Performed on a transverse section of the fetal skull at the level of the CSP, thalami, midline echo, and complete symmetrical cranium (see Fig. 25.16). The ultrasound's calipers are positioned perpendicular to the midline from the outer aspect of the upper parietal bone to the inner aspect of the opposite side.

Head circumference (HC)
Measured on the same section as the BPD. A trace is performed around the outer aspect of the cranium.

Abdominal circumference (AC)
A transverse section measured at the level of the stomach and intrahepatic portion of the umbilical vein (see Fig. 25.17). It is used in the third trimester to assess growth and to estimate fetal weight.

Femur length (FL)

A full-length view of the femur is obtained and calipers placed at each end (see Fig. 25.18). BPD and FL should correspond.

Adjunct to amniocentesis

Ultrasound is used pre-, post-, and often during amniocentesis and other invasive procedures. Pre-procedure it is used to assess fetal position, the location of the placenta, and to locate an accessible pool of amniotic fluid. Needle insertion and guidance can be imaged in real time using ultrasound.

Raised maternal serum alphafetoprotein (MSAFP)

Alphafetoprotein is produced by the fetal liver and reaches a peak in amniotic fluid at 16–18 weeks and in maternal blood at 32 weeks. It may be used as part of a screening test for fetal abnormalities. A raised MSAFP should result in a detailed scan of fetal anatomy.

Causes of raised MSAFP include:
- Neural tube defects—anencephaly, spina bifida, encephalocele.
- Abdominal wall defects.
- Gastrointestinal tract abnormalities.
- Other abnormalities, e.g., cleft palate.
- Wrong dates.
- Twins.
- Fetal demise.

Third trimester ultrasound

Indications include:
- Small for dates.
- Large for dates.
- Fetal distress.
- Vaginal bleeding.

Small for dates

The fetus may be small for dates because of incorrect dates and gestation being less than expected, difficulty in assessing gestation from palpation due to obesity of the mother, intrauterine growth retardation (IUGR), and reduced amniotic fluid (oligohydramnios).

IUGR

A fetus has IUGR when it is below the tenth centile for weight at any given gestational age or is less than 2.5 kg at 36 weeks. It is important to differentiate between a baby that is small for dates but normal, and one that is growth retarded. There are two main forms of IUGR:
- *Symmetrical*: The entire fetus is smaller than normal. Common causes include chromosomal abnormality, intrauterine viral infection, chronic maternal illness, or drug intake (smoking, alcohol). The diagnosis requires accurate dating at an early stage (first trimester or 18–22 week scan) and third trimester serial measurements of fetal head and trunk. Common measurements are HC and AC. Symmetrical IUGR will show a progressive fall off in growth for both parameters over time when compared to normal tables.
- *Asymmetrical*: The fetal trunk is small but the head is normal in size (brain sparing). It is caused by placental insufficiency. HC/AC ratio is needed to confirm the diagnosis (rule out hydrocephalus as another cause of high HC/AC—a low ratio may indicate microcephaly).

Oligohydramnios

Oligohydramnios is defined as a fluid pool less than 2 cm in depth. Causes include renal anomalies such as renal agenesis (check for the presence of the fetal bladder—excludes renal agenesis), neural tube defects and premature rupture of the membranes (US is useful in not only showing reduced fluid but also the size of the fetus, and whether a fetal anomaly is present. An anomaly with an associated polyhydramnios may have caused the membranes to rupture).

Large for dates

The causes include polyhydramnios, multiple gestation, macrosomia, incorrect dates, and uterine masses.

Polyhydramnios

Polyhydramnios is defined as a fluid pool greater than 8 cm.

Causes of polyhydramnios
• Fetal abnormalities affecting the gastrointestinal tract and the CNS (if swallowing mechanism affected)
• Skeletal and abdominal wall defects
• Diabetic pregnancy
• Multiple gestation
• Fetal hydrops
• Infections (toxoplasmosis and rubella)

Fig. 15.2 Causes of polyhydramnios.

Causes of polyhydramnios are outlined in Figure 15.2.

Multiple gestation

Problems associated with multiple pregnancies include IUGR, polyhydramnios, preterm delivery, and placenta previa. There is an increased incidence of fetal abnormality, particularly with monozygotic twins.

Macrosomia

Macrosomia is defined as a baby larger than 4 kg at birth, and this can cause problems during delivery. There is an association with maternal diabetes. The diagnosis is made with serial AC measurements. There may be associated polyhydramnios.

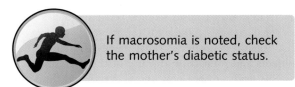
If macrosomia is noted, check the mother's diabetic status.

Incorrect dates

A mother presenting late in pregnancy may actually be at a later gestation than menstrual dates suggest.

Uterine masses

The presence of fibroids may cause uterine enlargement. US will demonstrate a solid mass within the uterine wall. Occasionally, fibroids may change in appearance as a result of cystic degeneration or bleeding (red degeneration). Scan should also check for maternal ovarian masses, which are predominantly cystic.

Fetal hydrops

This is characterized on US by fetal ascites, skin and scalp edema, pleural effusion, pericardial effusion, and polyhydramnios. If the placenta is thickened, Rhesus incompatibility (immune hydrops) is the likely cause. Other causes (non-immune hydrops) include fetal cardiac and chest abnormalities, infections (toxoplasmosis, rubella), and chromosomal disease.

Fetal distress

The fetus may be at risk of distress or death due to conditions such as:
- Maternal—chronic hypertension, pre-eclampsia, diabetes mellitus, and drug addiction.
- Fetal—presence of abnormality.
- Placental—insufficiency or fetal abruption.
- Previous history of stillbirth or distress.

Close monitoring of the fetus and its environment is essential to detect early signs of distress. Methods of detecting early distress include:
- *Biophysical profile*: A score is attributed to each of the following as observed over a 30-minute US scan: fetal breathing, fetal tone, fetal movement, amniotic fluid volume, and fetal heart rate. Total possible score is 10. Some centers have also assessed the placenta for signs of early maturity.
- *Umbilical artery Doppler*: The umbilical artery is sampled using Doppler US to obtain a waveform trace. The diastolic portion of the waveform is related to vascular resistance in the placenta. Increased resistance will cause decreased, absent, or reversed diastolic flow. Often the ratio of peak systolic to end diastolic is used to quantify this, i.e., the resistance index (RI). Abnormal findings on umbilical artery Doppler are associated with a poor outcome for the fetus.

Fetal death may occur in utero. US findings will vary depending on time since death (Fig. 15.3).

Vaginal bleeding

Placenta previa is defined as a placenta that partially or totally covers the internal os and is usually identified on the 18–22 week scan as a low-lying placenta. Most low-lying placentas identified on these early scans do not present as previa because of subsequent placental 'migration.' Separation from the myometrium may cause vaginal bleeding. Transabdominal US (with an empty bladder) will show previa. A full bladder may give the false impression of previa by compressing the cervix and making it appear longer. Vaginal scanning can be used to demonstrate the lower uterine segment if TAS is undiagnostic.

Placental abruption is caused by all, or some, of the placenta separating from the myometrium before delivery. Major abruptions are diagnosed clinically; the role of US is to determine fetal viability. Minor abruptions appear as an echopoor mass (clot) between the placenta and the myometrium. Amniotic fluid may contain echoes representing blood. Bleeding may also occur in the subchorionic portion of the placenta (marginal bleed) or within the placental tissue (intraplacental bleed).

Ultrasound findings in fetal death
• No evidence of fetal cardiac activity
• Absent fetal movement
• Skin edema
• Overlapping of skull bones (Spalding's sign)
• Biparietal diameter will decrease on subsequent scans
• Abnormal fetal position
• Fetal trunk appears collapsed

Fig. 15.3 Ultrasound findings in fetal death.

Case conference

A 28-year-old lady presents at 21 weeks' gestation with a raised maternal serum alphafetoprotein (MSAFP) as part of a routine biochemical analysis. Due to the increased incidence of fetal abnormality with raised MSAFP (in particular neural tube defects), a fetal anomaly scan was organized.

Ultrasound scan
Sagittal views of the fetus confirm viability with normal to increased fetal movement. Fetal trunk and limbs are identified but absence of the cranial vault is noted. Coronal views of the fetal face demonstrate a characteristic 'frogs' eyes' appearance. Transverse view for BPD again showed absence of bony skull (acrania) and cerebral hemispheres. The appearances are consistent with anencephaly.

The patient was referred for a tertiary level scan in the fetal medicine center and for counselling. The provisional diagnosis of anencephaly is confirmed.

PRINCIPLES OF RADIOLOGY

16. **Ionizing Radiation Studies**   87

17. **Non-ionizing Radiation Techniques**   91

18. **Nuclear Medicine**   93

16. Ionizing Radiation Studies

Radiology, or medical imaging, is a rapidly diversifying and increasingly pivotal discipline within medicine. Multiple imaging modalities are available. Some, e.g., CT, involve irradiation of the patient, and others, notably magnetic resonance and ultrasound, do not (Fig. 16.1).

Both the clinician and the radiologist involved in a patient's care should act to minimize any dose of ionizing radiation—the clinician through requesting appropriate investigations based on clinical acumen, and the radiologist in choosing the most appropriate imaging modality to gain the necessary information to aid diagnosis and management.

This section considers the phenomena involved in the generation of radiological images. The terminology used to describe findings is dependent on the imaging method used (see Fig. 16.1).

Conventional radiology

Production of x-rays

X-rays form part of the electromagnetic spectrum and are produced by heating a tungsten filament (the cathode) inside an evacuated tube (a vacuum). Electrons liberated from the cathode are focused on to an anode by creating a large potential difference between the two. X-ray photons are released from the anode by this electron bombardment. The casing of the x-ray tube absorbs most of the radiation, but a small proportion escapes through a window in the tube. This beam of radiation can be passed through the human body and detected by a photographic film (or digital imaging system). This film is sandwiched between two fluorescent screens. X-rays cause the emission of light from the screens and this light causes blackening of the film's emulsion once developed.

Radiographic appearances

It is possible to differentiate four separate tissues on radiographs because of their differential absorption of the x-ray beam (Fig. 16.2). All soft tissues, except fat, absorb the same amount of x-ray radiation and therefore appear the same shade of gray. Fat absorbs slightly less radiation than other soft tissues, and therefore looks a little darker. Bones absorb most radiation and therefore appear white, while air absorbs least and looks black. The fifth category is artefact, e.g., metallic foreign bodies, which appear as intense white foci on the radiograph.

Frontal chest radiograph (PA and AP projections)

The frontal chest radiograph is the most commonly requested radiological examination. The indications are diverse, but dyspnea, chest pain, and hemoptysis are common reasons for request.

Technically, the radiograph should be well centered with the medial borders of the clavicle equidistant from the spinous processes (see Fig. 19.1). A good inspiratory effort should be made, confirmed by identifying 10 ribs posteriorly at the level of the mid-clavicular line (see Fig. 19.2). It is mandatory to check the patient details and confirm that the name and the date of the examination are correct. Nipple markers can be useful (see Fig. 19.3).

When reviewing a chest film, a scheme of 'review areas' is indicated to ensure that all parts of the film are examined (Fig. 16.3).

Areas to review on the chest radiograph include:
- The cardiac silhouette
- The mediastinum
- The lung fields
- The costophrenic angles
- The diaphragm.

Lateral chest radiograph

The lateral chest radiograph may be useful for localizing, within the chest, a focal lesion (e.g., tumor) or artefact (e.g., pacing wires). One radiological maxim is that a pulmonary lesion not identified on the frontal chest radiograph is most unlikely to be seen on a lateral film. It should not be considered an alternative pulmonary imaging technique.

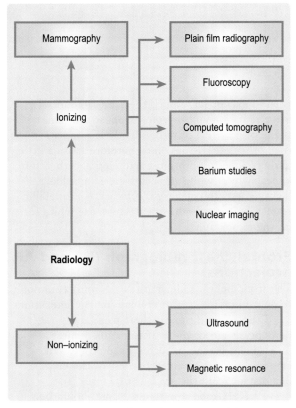

Fig. 16.1 Terminology of imaging modalities.

Appearance of plain radiographs	
Color	Tissue/artefact
Black	Gas
Dark grey	Fat
Grey	Soft tissues (except fat)
White	Bone
Intense white	Metallic objects

Fig. 16.2 Appearance on plain radiographs.

e.g., pneumoperitoneum, or bowel displacement by organomegaly. Renal or biliary calcification can also be demonstrated, as may bony pathology affecting the lower ribs, lumbar spinal column, and the pelvis.

Spinal radiographs
Spinal radiographs are typically requested to exclude trauma or arthropathy of the vertebral bone and joint architecture. Typically frontal and lateral (orthogonal) views are performed.

Cervical spine
At the cervical level, dedicated 'odontoid views' are also used. Check for visibility of all seven cervical vertebrae and the upper border of the first thoracic vertebral body. Check the vertebral alignment and the disc spacing. Check the arcs (alignment of the anterior and posterior vertebral margins and the spinolaminar line), the width of the paravertebral soft tissues and the shape of the prepharyngeal space.

 A C-spine *cannot* be cleared unless all seven cervical vertebrae and the first thoracic vertebra are seen.

Thoracic and lumbar spine
The main indications for these radiographs are back pain and following trauma. It is important to perform orthogonal (anterior and lateral) views. Check the vertebral alignment and the disc spacing, and the presence of pedicles (on the anterior view). Examine the apophyseal and the facet joints.

Apical chest radiograph
The apical radiograph is very useful in evaluating the upper aspects of each lung. This region is partially obscured by the clavicles and the upper ribs on the standard frontal chest radiograph. An apical view permits a clearer view of this region.

Abdominal radiograph
The supine abdominal film is commonly requested for the investigation of non-specific abdominal pain (Fig. 16.4).

Areas to review on the abdominal radiograph include:
- Bowel gas pattern (intraluminal gas)
- Extraluminal gas
- Vertebral column and pelvis.

Features to look for
The bowel should be evaluated to exclude gaseous distension of the small and/or large bowel and evidence of extraluminal air,

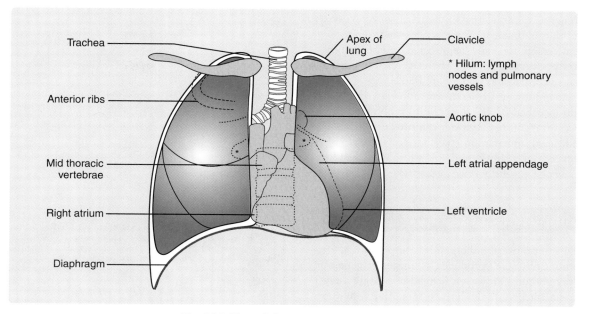

Fig. 16.3 Normal chest x-ray gross structures.

Limb x-rays

These are usually indicated to evaluate bone or joint pathology. Again orthogonal views are indicated. For symptomatology related to a bone, the joint at either end of that bone should be included on the radiograph.

Orthopedic radiographs usually require two views taken at right angles to each other. These are called orthogonal views.

Gastrointestinal imaging studies

The most common gastrointestinal (GI) contrast used is barium sulphate, which is completely inert but absorbs radiation very effectively. Different physical preparations of barium are used and in different concentrations depending on the study type, e.g., spherical molecules, considerably diluted, for small bowel studies, and small spikes of highly concentrated barium for upper GI studies. These latter molecules adhere to the esophageal and gastric mucosa, allowing excellent mucosal definition, particularly if used with an effervescent, gas-producing powder, or insufflated air (e.g., barium enema).

On occasion, e.g., if a gastrointestinal perforation is suspected, water-soluble contrast such as gastrograffin or iopamidol is used. This is because barium within the mediastinal space or peritoneal cavity is highly toxic, unlike the water-soluble media. They do, however, lack fine detail resolution and their role is chiefly to exclude obstruction and perforation.

Urography

Low osmolar water-soluble contrast such as iopamidol is injected intravenously and is filtered by the renal

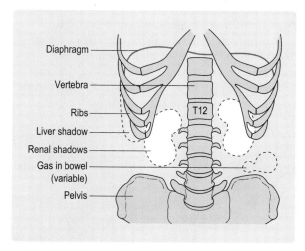

Fig. 16.4 Normal abdominal x-ray gross structures.

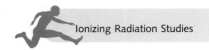

glomeruli, accumulating in the renal collecting system, and thus outlining it. Static images are taken to demonstrate the early 'nephrogram' phase, and the later pyelographic phase, when the renal calyces, pelvis, ureters, and bladder are filled.

As in all forms of contrast radiology, the control film (see Fig. 22.16), i.e., the film obtained prior to contrast administration, can provide valuable additional information (see Fig. 22.16), e.g., presence of a subtle renal calculus, and should always be carefully reviewed.

Fig. 16.5 Attenuation values on CT.

Computed tomography

Like conventional radiography, computed tomography (CT) produces its images by generating x-ray photons. However, instead of a single x-ray screen/film, multiple detectors and the x-ray tube rotate inside the ring (gantry), which surrounds the patient. Modern scanners use a helical technique whereby the patient advances through the gantry as it rotates, acquiring a volume of data. Ultrafast, helical multidetector (multislice) CT scanners allow very rapid scanning of body areas (e.g., thorax in 10 seconds). Multiplanar reconstructions allow superb three-dimensional images to be created.

The CT image is divided into picture elements (pixels) corresponding to a block of tissue (voxel) within the patient. Each pixel has an attenuation value (shade of gray) that depends on the corresponding voxel's composition. The attenuation value is measured in 'Hounsfield units' (HU). Air is typically −1000 HU; fat −50 HU; water 0 HU; soft tissue 30–80 HU; and bone +500 HU (Fig. 16.5). Metallic implants are +1000 HU.

It is important to remember that the radiation dose to the patient following CT scanning is considerable. For instance, helical CT of the chest produces a radiation dose of about 400 chest x-rays!

CT accounts for 15% of imaging but 75% of medical radiation exposure in the US.

Interventional radiology

This now comprises a very significant component of medical imaging, and spans the disciplines of diagnosis and therapy. Interventional procedures cover a wide spectrum. They can be divided into those procedures that access a vessel or tube (e.g., cerebro- or cardiovascular, biliary or urological) and those that access a pathological lesion directly via the shortest percutaneous route (e.g., abscess drainage, tumor or nodal biopsy).

Those procedures that access a vessel or tube employ the modified Seldinger technique. Following initial puncture of the vessel with a needle, a guide wire is advanced along the lumen. The needle is withdrawn and a catheter advanced over the wire. Following correct catheter placement, subsequent delivery of angioplasty balloons, expandable stents, occluding coils, glues, or microspheres are all feasible.

- List non-ionizing radiation imaging modalities.
- What factors must be considered when technically assessing the quality of a chest x-ray?
- What are orthogonal views?
- What is a Hounsfield unit?
- List the review areas on a chest x-ray assessment.
- Explain the modified Seldinger technique.

17. Non-ionizing Radiation Techniques

Ultrasound

Ultrasound has no ionizing radiation associated with it and there are no practical safety aspects within the diagnostic power range. Diagnostic ultrasound waves are produced by using an electromagnetic field to produce alteration of the physical shape of piezoelectric crystals (a transducer) within the probe. This shape alteration causes emission of the sound waves. These high frequency waves, having been emitted by the probe, enter the body, are reflected back by internal structures and are detected by the same probe. The diagnostic frequency range is between 2 and 20 MHz. Various probes of different frequencies are available depending on the structures being imaged.

The scanned region is represented on a monitor screen by shades of gray, the shade describing the tissue's echogenicity. Fatty tissue is slightly brighter (hyperechoic) than surrounding tissue, while fluid is completely black (anechoic). In modern real-time ultrasound machines, multiple transducer elements are arranged in rows (arrays) within the probe. These allow an instantaneous image that can be updated by altering the frame rate, usually a range of between 20 and 200 frames per second. Ultrasound is a dynamic investigation and observing the moving image is often more valuable than evaluating the static printed scans.

Ultrasound cannot penetrate gas or bone. Overlying ribs and aerated lung therefore prevent imaging of deeper structures.

Doppler ultrasound

The Doppler effect describes alteration in sound frequency caused by movement between the sound source and the observer, e.g., the changing pitch of a motorcycle engine as it passes a stationary spectator. In ultrasound, the sound source (and 'listener') is the probe. A dual function probe transducer produces what is known as 'pulsed wave Doppler.' Approximately 95% of the probe time is in the listening mode.

Movement of red blood cells relative to the probe produces alteration in frequency. This frequency change can be displayed as a spectral trace, a color, or an audible signal.

Common indications for Doppler ultrasound would include peripheral vascular examinations, particularly in lower limb diagnosis of deep venous thrombosis and venous insufficiency. Other indications include carotid Doppler examination in TIA/stroke/neurological disturbance, abdominal Doppler imaging in portal hypertension, Budd–Chiari syndrome, and fetal–maternal medicine imaging of the umbilical vessels.

Abdominal ultrasound scan

Indications include abdominal pain, jaundice, renal dysfunction or obstruction, abdominal mass, or abdominal distension.

What to look for

Ultrasound examination of the abdomen and pelvis is a methodical examination of the gallbladder, biliary tree, liver, spleen, pancreas, kidneys, aorta, vena cava and urinary bladder, and, in the female patient, the adnexa, i.e., the uterus, cervix, and ovaries.

Patients referred for hepatobiliary ultrasound should be fasted for at least 4 hours. Those requiring pelvic ultrasound should have a full bladder.

Cardiac ultrasound

Echocardiography uses both a real-time image and M (movement) mode ultrasound. M mode ultrasound is a continuously moving amplitude (A mode) waveform. In A mode, the height of the 'spike' relates to its echointensity, and its position on the horizontal axis, its depth (like sonar).

Cardiac ultrasound is used to assess the heart chamber size, valve and wall motion. Common indications would be valve disease, septal defects,

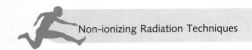
cardiomyopathy, cardiac failure, assessment of systolic function, and quantification of pericardial effusion.

Magnetic resonance imaging

The physics of magnetic resonance (MR) depend on the fact that the nucleus of every hydrogen atom in every water molecule has magnetic properties. This is because they are charged particles, protons, which spin. If an external magnetic field is applied, these protons align themselves to that field, wobbling about the field axis with a motion known as 'precession.' When a second magnetic field, in the form of a radiofrequency (RF) pulse, is applied at right angles to the first, the protons' vector alters to become perpendicular to the external magnetic field, and they gain energy and spin synchronously. This is known as being 'in phase.'

Once the RF pulse stops, the protons do two things: firstly they shed their extra newly acquired energy back to the surrounding chemical lattice.

This is known as T1 relaxation. Secondly, they stop spinning synchronously. This asynchronous dephasing is known as T2 relaxation.

As a rule, T1 images produce good anatomical detail, whereas T2 images are more representative of tissue pathology. Inversion recovery (IR) or fat suppression sequences highlight areas of fluid, both normal (e.g., CSF) and pathological (e.g., focal areas of infection, trauma, inflammation, and malignancy).

MRI was initially used for the evaluation of the central nervous system, i.e., the brain and spinal cord (see Fig. 24.1). More recently multiple and diverse applications of MRI have been realized. In neuroradiological imaging, perfusion and diffusion imaging has evolved in the evaluation of strokes and of focal brain lesions and tumour recurrence, respectively. Improved resolution and faster imaging times have resulted in MR being used to image the biliary tree (magnetic resonance cholangiopancreatography, MRCP), and the central and peripheral vascular systems (magnetic resonance angiography, MRA).

- When might Doppler ultrasound be used?
- What patient preparation might be necessary before ultrasound of the abdomen?
- What is the difference between T1 and T2 weighted MR imaging?
- What should be checked with a patient before undergoing an MRI scan?

18. Nuclear Medicine

Nuclear medicine is a specialty that produces images of function rather than anatomy. Tiny amounts of radiopharmaceuticals (usually of the order of micrograms) permit imaging without interference in the body's physiological and biochemical processes. Radiopharmaceuticals are labelled with radioactive isotopes that decay to produce gamma photons (like high energy x-rays).

Different types of gamma cameras are used to detect these gamma photons and produce an image of the radiopharmaceutical distribution within the body. Many different radiopharmaceuticals and radioisotopes are utilized to image different functions in various body organs.

The quantity (dose) of radiopharmaceutical used is measured in megaBecquerels or MBq (1 Becquerel is one decay per second). The dose is a balance between image quality, from lots of gamma photons, and minimum radiation effects within the patient.

Average US annual background radiation is 2.2 mSV.

Nuclear imaging produces functional rather than structural images.

The amount of radiation absorbed by the patient is called the effective dose (ED) and is measured in milliSieverts (mSv). Generally, the longer the half-life of a radioisotope, the higher its ED.

Isotopes

Isotopes are described by their atomic weight, e.g., Tc^{99m} (technetium). Doses are given as megaBecquerels (MBq) and the effective dose (ED) as milliSieverts (mSv).

$Technetium^{99m}$ is the most common radioisotope used in nuclear medicine because of its characteristics. The short (6 hour) half-life allows labelling of the radiopharmaceutical, transfer to the imaging department, injection of the patient and imaging, but within 24 hours very little radioactivity is present in the patient (Fig. 18.1). Gamma photons of a specific and single energy level are produced and are detected by the gamma camera.

$Indium^{111}$ is usually used when images need to be obtained beyond 24 hours. This is important if uptake of the radiopharmaceutical is slow or if the function being imaged is intermittent. This may be used for the detection of an abscess or in assessing the extent and distribution of inflammatory bowel disease using radiolabelled white cells.

$Iodine^{123}$ is often used when new pharmaceuticals are produced because the chemistry of labelling compounds with iodine is often simpler.

Single photon emission computed tomography (SPECT)

Radioactive decay from tissues surrounding the organ of interest can reduce the image contrast, and activity in adjacent viscera or blood vessels reduces the ability to quantify the core activity. Tomography addresses both these issues. In single photon emission computed tomography (SPECT) studies, a conventional gamma camera rotates 360° around the patient. Standard isotopes such as technetium are used. A single photon from each nuclear disintegration is identified.

Positron emission tomography (PET)

Positron emission tomography (PET) is a relatively new and rapidly expanding nuclear medicine technique that utilizes the emission of positrons by specific isotopes. Such elements contain excess

Technetium - 99M for VQ scanning

Albumin

Technetium

Absorbed dose	70 MBq
Equivalent dose	1 mSv
Effective dose	1 mSv
Half-life	6 hours
Energy level of Gamma Ray	140 KeV
Equivalent to CXR	50
Equivalent to background radiation	6 months

Fig. 18.1 Typical radioisotope.

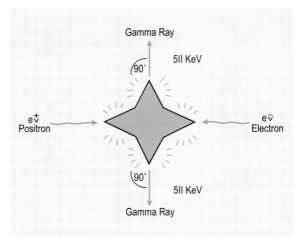

Gamma Ray

5ll KeV

90°

e^+_v Positron

e^-_v Electron

90°

5ll KeV

Gamma Ray

Fig. 18.2 Positron emission tomography annihilation event.

protons that decay to form a neutron and a positron (antimatter). A positron is a positively charged electron. The positron travels approximately 2 mm beyond the atom and collides with an electron. The collision, known as annihilation, results in the formation of two gamma rays with a specific energy of 511 keV (Fig. 18.2). These two gamma rays travel in opposite directions and are absorbed by two detectors located around the patient. The PET scanner's computer system can subsequently localize the site of the annihilation event within the patient.

The most frequently used isotope in clinical practice is fluorodeoxyglucose[18] (FDG). This radiopharmaceutical images glucose uptake via glucose transporter proteins. These are overexpressed in most common malignancies. Such tumors are said to be 'glucose avid' and absorb the glucose analogue, FDG. When subsequent positron emission begins within the tumor, detectors localize its position within the body. It is therefore possible to identify sites of active or recurrent disease, and to differentiate them from scar tissue or fibrosis. The disadvantages of PET are that not all tumors are glucose avid, the isotopes are short

lived (FDG, 2 hours), and a cyclotron is required to produce them.

PET–CT combines PET (functional imaging) with CT (structural imaging) to give the best results.

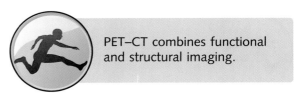

PET–CT combines functional and structural imaging.

Specific isotope studies

Lung scanning (ventilation perfusion, V/Q scans)

Lung scanning is almost always performed to identify a pulmonary embolus (PE). An acute PE disrupts the blood supply to part of the lung without interfering with ventilation. Isotope scanning identifies this area that is ventilated but not perfused—a mismatch—and permits the diagnosis to be made. Segmental areas of absent perfusion with normal ventilation are seen in PE.

Perfusion scanning is performed with technetium labelled to macroaggregates of albumin (MAA). These have a diameter of 100 μm and

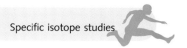

image the perfusion at the pre-alveolar arteriolar level. The dose is 70 MBq (ED = 1 mSv).

Ventilation imaging may be performed with a variety of isotopes, e.g., krypton Kr^{81m}, eluted from a rubidium generator. The dose of krypton is 6000 MBq, but because the half-life is only 13 seconds, the ED is only 0.2 mSv. Alternatives include Xenon, Xe^{133} (400 MBq, ED = 0.4 mSv) or technetium labelled aerosols, e.g., DTPA (80 MBq, ED = 0.4 mSV). Note that the ED of all ventilation scans is very small.

Bone scanning

Bone scanning is performed with technetium methylene diphosphonate, $Tc^{99m}MDP$ (and other similar diphosphonates). The dose is 555 MBq and the ED is 1 mSv. This radiopharmaceutical images osteoblastic activity and the deposition of hydroxyapatite into the osteoid matrix.

There are two chief forms of bone scanning: static and dynamic. With static studies, images are acquired 2 hours after IV administration. This is principally performed to stage malignancy, establish the presence of fractures or identify metabolic bone disease. In dynamic studies, images are acquired immediately at the time of injection (flow phase), 5–10 minutes later (pool phase), and at the 2 hour (static) phase. This type of bone scan is used to establish the presence of osteomyelitis.

Kidney
Renal structure

This is evaluated (as is renal function) using a technetium labelled DMSA (dimercaptosuccinic acid) scan. The dose is 80 MBq and the ED is 1.0 mSv. This radiopharmaceutical images the amount of functioning proximal convoluted tubular cells and is used to image acute and chronic pyelonephritis. This allows for assessment of differential renal function.

Renal excretion

There is a choice of two isotopes: Tc-labelled MAG-3 (mercaptoacetyltriglycene), which is actively excreted at the proximal convoluted tubule, or DTPA (diethylene triamine pentacetic acid), which is filtered at the glomerulus. ED is 0.7 mSv. These scans assess how efficiently the urine produced by the kidney drains into the ureter and bladder.

Thyroid scanning

Thyroid studies image the function of the sodium–iodide symporter chain. The isotope chiefly used in imaging the thyroid is technetium pertechnetate $(Tc^{99m}O_4^-)$ with a dose of 80 MBq (ED = 1 mSv). Thyroid isotope studies can also be performed with an iodine isotope, I^{123}, with a dose of 20 MBq (ED = 3 mSv). Note that the effective dose is larger for I^{123} even though a smaller dose is given. This is because of its longer half-life.

Parathyroid scanning

Isotopes used are technetium pertechnetate, with a dose of 70 MBq, and Tc^{99m} MIBI (methoxyisobutyl isonitrile). MIBI is taken up by both the thyroid and the parathyroid adenoma whereas technetium is taken up by only the thyroid. As MIBI is not taken up by the normal parathyroid, it is possible to subtract one image from the other and localize parathyroid adenomas.

Lymphangiography

In this test, the transport of extracellular proteins through lymphatics of an affected limb is imaged. The isotope used is technetium human albumin nanocolloid. The dose is 40 MBq and the ED is 0.5 mSv. The study is typically performed to evaluate lower limb lymphatics. Isotope is injected into the web space between the toes. Inguinal nodes are imaged between 1 and 3 hours later, but in diseased states may be imaged at up to 24 hours.

Cardiac imaging

This test images the perfusion of the oxygenated functioning myocardial tissue and depends on the radiopharmaceutical $(Tc^{99m}$ MIBI) being trapped in the functioning mitochondria. The dose is 400 MBq with an ED of 0.5 mSv.

Thallium (Tl^{201}), which was previously the traditionally used myocardial radiopharmaceutical, is a potassium analogue that images the perfusion of cardiac muscle with a functioning, energy-dependent Na/K ATPase system.

Myocardial perfusion imaging may help distinguish necrotic from ischemic myocardium.

Adrenal medullary imaging

Adrenal imaging is performed with I^{123} MIBG (meta-iodo-benzyl-guanidine). This is a guanethidine analogue taken up by cells which produce adrenaline, e.g., adrenergic nerve cells and the adrenal medulla. The dose is 400 MBq with an ED of 6 mSv. This is used in the investigation of a phaeochromocytoma, in particular localization of extra-adrenal lesions.

White cell imaging

This can be performed with technetium HMPAO (Ceretec) with a dose of 200 MBq or with indium tropolone with a dose of 20–40 MBq (ED = 9 mSv). The radiopharmaceutical is used to label the patient's own white blood cells derived from a large (120 mL) blood sample that is subsequently reinjected. This scan images granulocyte migration from the intravascular to the extravascular space and is used to image infection and inflammatory bowel disease.

Red cell imaging

This is usually performed with technetium and sometimes indium labelled red cells. Red cell imaging identifies very small amounts of blood loss into the gastrointestinal tract. The camera detects movement of labelled red blood cells from the intravascular space into the gut lumen.

Blood loss is evaluated with images taken at 1, 2, 6 and 24 hours following the injection. The dose is 400 MBq. Technetium labelled sulphur colloid (dose 80 MBq) can also be used. Both techniques image active bleeding during the study and can detect a bleeding rate down to 0.5 mL per minute.

Liver and spleen imaging

Any colloid is useful; for example, technetium sulphur colloid, technetium antimony sulphide colloid, and technetium tin colloid. Spleen imaging is with technetium labelled heat denatured red blood cells. Dose is 40 MBq with an ED of 2 mSv. These are now rarely used.

Biliary imaging

Biliary imaging is performed using technetium hepatoiminodiacetic acid (HIDA). The dose is 80–120 MBq with an ED of 1 mSv. The HIDA compounds image the drainage of bile from the liver, through the biliary tree, and into the duodenum.

Chronic infection

This can be imaged with gallium (Ga^{67}). The dose is 150 MBq and the ED is 12 mSv. Ga^{67} is an iron analogue, and iron is a requirement of many bacteria. Gallium is also taken up by sarcoid and many tumors.

Principal radionuclides used in medical imaging				
Element	Radionuclide	Half-life	Energy level	Use
Technetium	Tc^{99m}	6 hours	140 keV	Organ imaging
Gallium	Ga^{67}	7–8 hours	90–93 keV 185 keV 300 keV	Localization of neoplasms, abscesses and sarcoid
Krypton	Kr^{81m}	13.5 seconds	190 keV	Lung ventilation imaging
Indium	In^{111}	2.8 days	171 keV 250 keV	Cell labelling and CSF imaging, longer studies generally
Iodine	I^{123}	13.3 hours	160 keV	Use in thyroid and adrenal imaging (MIBG)
Iodine	I^{131}	8.1 days	610 keV 360 keV	Use in thyroid treatment (hyperthyroidism and thyroid cancer)
Thallium	Tl^{201}	74 hours	70 keV	Myocardial imaging

Fig. 18.3 Principal radionuclides used in medical imaging.

Attach addressograph Label or print in CAPITALS

Hospital No: ___BR 645268___

Full Name: _____

Address: _____

_____

DOB: _22/11/54_ Tel No: _____

Ward/Dept: _6F_ Consultant: ___WEEKLEY___

Departmental Use Only

ID Check

Name ☐   Date of Appointment: _____

Address ☐   Time: _____ Room No: _____

DOB ☐   **Pregnancy Status** (delete as applicable)
Pregnant / Not Pregnant **LMP** / /
Breast feeding: Yes / No

Summary of clinical history (50) 25 year-history Rheumatoid disease. Two years on Methotrexate. No previous chest disease 6/12 ↑ SOB, dry cough. Exercise tolerance 100 yards o/E Bilateral basal fine inspiratory crepitations

Mobility Status
Bed ☑ Portable ☐
Walking ☐ Chair ☐

What clinical queries should this study answer? Interstitial lung Disease?

Infection Status
MRSA ⊕

Pressure Risk Score
NO RISK

For specialist examinations, please state known contra-indications. Nil Contraindications

Patient Category
NHS ☑ Private ☐ Category 2 ☐

All previous images must accompany patients.

Examination suggested: HRCT CHEST

Pregnant: Yes / No N/A
LMP / /

REFERRER:

Referrer (signature) _____ Name (printed) _____

Job title: CONS/SPR/SHO/JHO/NP/GP (please circle) Bleep/Contact No. _2064_ Date _24/11/2004_

All incomplete and illegible forms will be returned.

Fig. 18.4 X-ray request.

Tumor imaging

Octreotide is indium[111] labelled sandostatin. The dose is 185 MBq. The half life is 2–3 days. The octreotide images somatostatin receptors produced by many neuroendocrine tumors. Images are taken at 24 and 48 hours. It is useful in evaluating GI hormone tumors such as carcinoid, vipoma, and insulinoma.

The principal radionuclides used in medical imaging are outlined in Figure 18.3.

Radiation doses and requests

Statutory regulations, namely the Nuclear Regulatory Commission (NRC) 2000, require referrers, practitioners, and operators to limit the dose of diagnostic radiation to patients. Each exposure must be justified (Fig. 18.4).

The additional lifetime risk of acquiring a fatal cancer from the Earth's background radiation or a chest x-ray is 1 in a million. However, following an abdominal CT examination, the risk rises sharply to 1 in 2000. Conversely, the risk of acquiring a malignancy during one's lifetime is 1 in 3. Therefore the risk–benefit of an examination must always be considered. This is particularly pertinent if repeated imaging is required.

The Royal College of Radiologists has issued guidance for doctors in its booklet *Making the Best use of a Radiology Department* (5th edn, 2003). Reproduced below are two tables from this booklet (Figs 18.5, 18.6) illustrating the doses of common imaging investigations.

Typical effective doses from diagnostic medical exposure in the 2000s			
Diagnostic procedure	Typical effective doses (mSv)	Equivalent no. of chest x-rays	Equivalent period of background radiation
Limb/joint except hip	<0.01	<0.5	<1.5 days
Chest (PA film)	0.02	1	3 days
Skull	0.06	3	9 days
Thoracic spine	0.07	35	4 months
Lumbar spine	1.0	50	5 months
Hip	0.4	20	2 months
Pelvis	0.7	35	4 months
Abdomen	0.7	35	4 months
IVP	2.4	120	14 months
Barium swallow	1.5	75	8 months
Barium meal	2.6	130	15 months
Barium follow-through	3	150	16 months
Barium enema	7.2	360	3.2 years
CT head	2.0	100	10 months
CT chest	8	400	3.6 years
CT abdomen or pelvis	10	500	4.5 years
Lung ventilation (Xe^{133})	0.3	15	7 weeks
Lung perfusion (Tc^{99m})	1	50	6 months
Kidney (Tc^{99m})	1	50	6 months
Thyroid (Tc^{99m})	1	50	6 months
Bone (Tc^{99m})	4	200	1.8 years
Dynamic cardiac (Tc^{99m})	6	300	2.7 years
PET head (^{18}FDG)	5	250	2.3 years

Fig. 18.5 Typical effective doses from diagnostic medical exposure in the 2000s. (Reproduced with permission from the Royal College of Radiologists.)

Band classifications of the typical effective doses of ionizing radiation from common imaging procedures		
Band	Typical effective dose (mSv)	Examples
0	0	US, MRI
I	<1	CXR, XR limb, XR pelvis
II	1–5	IVP, XR lumbar spine, NM (e.g. skeletal scintigram) CT head and neck
III	6–10	CT chest or abdomen, NM (e.g. cardiac)
IV	>10	Extensive CT studies, some NM studies (e.g. PET)

Fig. 18.6 Band classification of the typical effective doses of ionizing radiation from common imaging procedures. (Reproduced with permission from the Royal College of Radiologists.)

Always consider radiation dose when requesting imaging investigations.

- In what unit is a radiopharmaceutical dose measured?
- What properties make technetium^{99m} a good radioisotope for clinical imaging?
- When might PET imaging be useful?
- What regulations govern the use of radiation in patients?
- What is the effective dose of a CT chest?

IMAGE GALLERY

19. Respiratory Imaging   103

20. Cardiac and Breast Imaging   113

21. Gastrointestinal Imaging   121

22. Abdominal Imaging   131

23. Orthopedic Imaging   139

24. Head and Neck Imaging   151

25. Pediatric Radiology   163

19. Respiratory Imaging

Fig. 19.1 Reference chest x-ray (CXR). All areas to be assessed • patient details • technical factors • cardiac silhouette • mediastinum • lungs • bones • soft tissues

a

b

Fig. 19.2 Normal CXR: (a) Poor inspiratory effort; (b) the same patient with normal inspiratory effort.

Fig. 19.4 CT chest: Section at the level of the right upper lobe bronchus (RULB).

Fig. 19.3 Female CXR: (a) With nipple shadows; (b) with nipple markers, showing their usefulness. These are used to differentiate nipple shadows from an intrapulmonary mass.

Fig. 19.5 VQ Scan: Pulmonary emboli. (a) Lung perfusion (b) lung ventilation. There are perfusion defects (*); ventilation scan normal, unmatched defect.

Fig. 19.7 Emphysema, CXR: Lungs overinflated • Greater than 10 ribs visible posteriorly • Flattened diaphragms • Enlarged central pulmonary arteries • Peripheral pruning.

Fig. 19.6 Surgical emphysema in polytrauma, CT scan: (a) chest; (b) abdomen. Air in the soft tissues (arrows) extends from the neck to the scrotum.

Fig. 19.9 Right apical tuberculosis, previous thoraco-plasty, CXR (*): Increased density ● Scarring ● Interstitial lung changes and volume loss.

Fig. 19.8 Bronchiectasis, (a) high-resolution CT scan, (b) CXR left lower lobe: Enlarged bronchi with crowding ● Bronchi visible to the extremity of lung field ● May be fluid levels within the bronchi ● May be associated conso-lidation ● May be associated interstitial lung disease.

Fig. 19.10 Bilateral pulmonary fibrosis, (a) high-resolution CT scan, (b) CXR: Subpleural location and basal predominance • Reticulonodular shadowing ('lines and dots' appearance) • Cardiac and diaphragmatic silhouette may be visible on x-ray.

Fig. 19.11 Lower lobe consolidation, CXR: (a) Right lower lobe (*); (b) left lower lobe. Loss of the right/left hemidiaphragm • Elevation of the diaphragm • Ipsilateral mediastinal shift.

107

Fig. 19.12 Pneumocystis jiroveci (formerly *P. carinii*) pneumonia, CXR: Initial interstitial pattern • Progression to air space change within 5 days • There are subtle perihilar interstitial markings that will progress, if untreated, to form consolidation.

Fig. 19.13 Pneumothorax, CXR: (a) Right side pre-drain; (b) chest drain in place. Note difference in transradiancy (blackness) between the two pre-drain lungs • Pre-drain collapsed lung edge identifiable (arrows) with tension, depression of diaphragm and contralateral mediastinal shift • Post-drain no lung edge visible, mediastinum and diaphragm in normal position.

Fig. 19.14 Cavitating right lung, CXR: Opacity seen within the lung • Central lucency within opacity, plus or minus fluid level.

Fig. 19.16 Left apical carcinoma, CXR: Increased-density apex (*) • Irregular margin, does not correspond to lobe • May be bulging of associated fissures • May be associated lymphadenopathy or metastatic disease • Associated rib erosion.

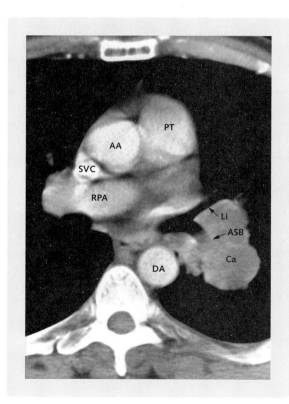

Fig. 19.15 Carcinoma of left lung, CT scan: Low attenuation mass adjacent to hilum, endobronchial compression, associated lymphadenopathy. (AA, ascending aorta; ASB, apical segmental; bronchus of the left lower lobe; Ca, carcinoma of the left lung; DA, descending aorta; Li, lingular bronchus; PT, pulmonary trunk; RPA, right pulmonary artery; SVC, superior vena cava.)

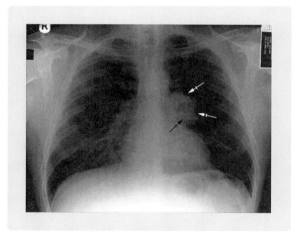

Fig. 19.17 Left hilar mass, CXR: Enlarged left hilum • May be associated consolidation and volume loss • Look for central lymphadenopathy • Look for pulmonary metastases • The hila, although at different levels, should normally be the same size and density.

Fig. 19.18 Sarcoidosis, CXR: Bilateral hilar lymphadenopathy ● May be right paratracheal lymphadenopathy (Garland's syndrome) ● Look for interstitial lung disease.

Fig. 19.20 Pulmonary embolus, (a) contrast-enhanced CT, (b) CXR: Large embolus seen within right pulmonary artery (arrows) ● Enlarged right pulmonary artery. (DA, descending aorta; AA, ascending aorta; SVC, superior vena cava; RPA, right pulmonary artery; PT, pulmonary trunk.)

Fig. 19.19 Right-sided mesothelioma, CXR: Nobulated pleural thickening with lobulated nature ● Lesion encircles right lung ● No volume loss.

Fig. 19.21 Left pleural effusion, erect CXR: Loss of left hemidiaphragm • Meniscus laterally at chest wall (arrows) • Lack of mediastinal movement indicates associated underlying lobe or collapse.

a

b

Fig. 19.22 Pulmonary metastases, (a) CXR, (b) CT: Multiple pulmonary nodules evident • Non-specific appearance • Patient history essential.

111

Fig. 19.23 Left upper lobe collapse, CXR: Decreased visibility of aortic knob, veil-like opacity, diaphragmatic elevation, and ipsilateral mediastinal elevation.

Fig. 19.25 Pectus excavatum, CXR: Cardiac silhouette displaces to the left, mimicking right middle lobe consolidation, heart shaped ribs • Diagnosis is confirmed by examining patient (not by performing lateral CXR).

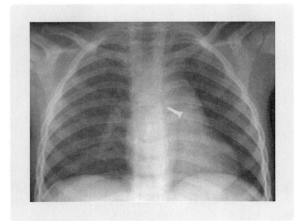

Fig. 19.24 Inhaled foreign body in left main bronchus, CXR: Foreign body may be visible • Initially overinflation of lung with diaphragmatic depression and contralateral mediastinal movement; later there is volume loss, diaphragmatic elevation, and ipsilateral mediastinal movement.

Fig. 19.26 Miliary tuberculosis, CXR: Fine opacities within both lungs • Appearance is non-specific so patient history essential.

Fig. 20.1 Internal carotid artery, carotid angiogram: Area of stenosis identified beyond the bifurcation of the carotid artery • Distal carotid vessel patent • External carotid artery patent.

Fig. 20.3 Atrial septal defect, CXR: Pulmonary plethora ± cardiomegaly • Small aortic knob • Aortic knob contour may or may not be normal.

Fig. 20.2 Left ventricular aneurysm, chest x-ray (CXR): Square shape to left ventricle (arrows) • May be cardiomegaly • Look for evidence of cardiac failure • May be ventricular calcification.

Fig. 20.4 Aortic coarctation, CXR: Notching identified ribs 4–10 (Dock's sign, arrows).

Fig. 20.5 Cardiac failure, CXR: The heart is enlarged • Increased pulmonary venous vascularity • Upper zone diversion • Kerley B lines • Pleural effusions • Air space consolidation in pulmonary edema.

Fig. 20.6 Left atrial enlargement, CXR: Cardiomegaly • Splaying of the carina (angle greater than 90°) • Left atrial appendage (LAA) enlargement (arrow) • Double atrial shadow • In this case the left atrial wall is calcified.

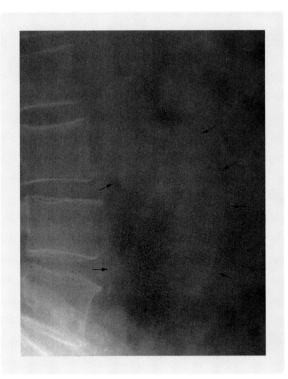

Fig. 20.7 Abdominal aortic aneurysm (arrows), lateral lumbar spine x-ray: Calcification of the aorta • Loss of aortic wall parallelism • Superior mesenteric artery if calcified provides good marker for the position of renal arteries.

Fig. 20.8 Aortic dissection, CT chest. (AA, ascending aortic arch; DA, descending aortic arch; F, dissection flap; O, esophagus; SVC, superior vena cava; T, trachea; VB, vertebral body.)

Fig. 20.10 Fibromuscular hyperplasia, renal artery angiogram: Beaded appearance to renal arteries.

Fig. 20.9 Right iliac artery, DSA: Pre-intervention irregularity and narrowing of the right external iliac artery • Post-intervention diameter of vessel restored • No significant stenosis • Check distal vessels remain patent • The radiologist will check no residual pressure gradient across the stent.

Fig. 20.11 Aortic stent placement, AXR: Stent appearance will vary according to manufacturer • Typically metallic lattice along the length of the aortic ± iliac arteries.

Fig. 20.12 Pericardial effusion, CXR: Heart significantly enlarged and has globular appearance • Diagnosis confirmed on echocardiography.

Fig. 20.13 Doppler spectral waveform: Normal external carotid artery.

Fig. 20.14 CT abdomen: Inferior vena caval filter (arrows).

Fig. 20.15 Left mastectomy, CXR: Different transparency of both lungs • Left breast shadow absent • Left hilar mass (arrows). Indicates recurrent disease.

Fig. 20.16 Mammogram, oblique view: Fibroadenoma with popcorn calcification.

Fig. 20.17 Ultrasound: Breast carcinoma.

Fig. 20.18 Mammograms, (a) oblique and (b) craniocaudal views: Spiculated breast carcinoma with lymphadenopathy and skin retraction.

Fig. 20.19 Mammogram, oblique view: Spiculated breast carcinoma.

Fig. 20.21 Mammogram, craniocaudal view: Branching calcification in keeping with carcinoma.

Fig. 20.20 Ultrasound: Breast abscess.

Fig. 20.22 Mammograms, (a) oblique and (b) craniocaudal views: Spiculated mass in keeping with a carcinoma.

Fig. 21.1 Achalasia, barium swallow: Dilated esophagus
• Smooth contour to walls • Tapers to a beak at distal end
• No shouldering of esophageal lesion.

Fig. 21.2 Achalasia, chest x-ray (CXR): Grossly widened mediastinum (arrows) • Distended, fluid-filled esophagus is seen in the midline (arrows), extending into the neck • Extends above level of aortic knob • Fluid level may be apparent • Signs of chronic aspiration may be apparent in lower lobes of lung • Typically a small gastric shadow on chest x-ray.

Fig. 21.3 Candidiasis, barium swallow: Multiple small filling defects • Irregular mucosa • Long segment involvement (continuous).

Fig. 21.4 Esophageal web, barium swallow: Usually situated at pharyngo-esophageal junction (C6 vertebra) • Thin, linear filling defect • Normally arises from anterior esophageal wall • Can be circumferential and multiple • In association with iron deficiency anemia and koilonychia known as Paterson–Brown Kelly (Plummer–Vinson) syndrome • Risk of development of esophageal malignancy.

Fig. 21.6 Esophageal varices, barium swallow: Multiple
• Long serpiginous filling defects.

Fig. 21.5 Corrosive (benign) stricture, barium swallow:
Long segment involvement • Smooth contour to stricture
when established (after acute incident) • Often proximal
dilatation of esophagus • With time may develop esophageal malignancy (see Fig. 21.7 for features) • Commonly
occurs in children from accidental ingestion of corrosive
liquid.

Fig. 21.7 Esophageal carcinoma, barium swallow: Short stricture • Loss of normal mucosa giving an irregular outline—note the shouldered margins of the tumor (barred arrows) and the irregular, narrowed mucosa (arrows) • With an irregular mucosa is the key finding of malignancy • Short shouldered lesion.

Fig. 21.8 Pharyngeal pouch, barium swallow: Pooling of barium in pharyngeal outpouching (*) • Occurs at Killian's dehiscence • Relative contraindication for endoscopy in 'dysphagia' patient • Disease of older patients (> 55 years of age).

Fig. 21.9 Pneumoperitoneum, erect CXR: Free air (*) under both hemidiaphragms (arrows) (L, liver; S, spleen) • Usually more on the right, interposed between the diaphragm and liver • Gastric 'air' bubble may obscure on the left side and may be mistaken for free air.

Fig. 21.12 Hiatus hernia, retrocardiac air-fluid level, CXR: Mediastinal soft tissue mass (*) ● Left lateral film will confirm the retrocardiac level ● Barium study will confirm the diagnosis.

Fig. 21.10 Pneumoperitoneum, Rigler's sign, supine CXR: The bowel wall is visible (arrows), because of gas within bowel lumen and peritoneum, latter seen as air within the fibers of the psoas muscle ● Pneumoperitoneum due to a gun-shot wound.

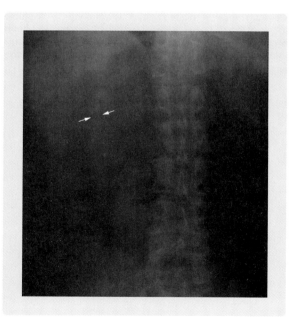

Fig. 21.11 Pneumoperitoneum falciform ligament sign, supine abdominal x-ray (AXR): Falciform ligament outlined by free gas (arrows) ● Extends from liver to umbilicus (umbilicus relates to L3).

Fig. 21.13 Gastric carcinoma, barium meal: Irregular appearance to mucosa ● Contracted lumen of stomach ● Differential diagnosis of a gastric lymphoma should be considered.

Fig. 21.14 Crohn's disease string sign (of Kantor), small bowel study: There is a well-defined strictured segment of small bowel in the ileum (arrows)—may be short, long, single or multiple • Rose thorn ulceration (due to deep fissured ulceration) • Bowel loop separation • Cobblestone appearance to mucosa.

Fig. 21.15 Small bowel obstruction, supine AXR: Centrally located dilated small bowel loops • Multiple loops of small bowel • Greater than 3 cm but less than 5 cm in diameter • Valvulae conniventes (mucosal markings across full width of bowel) • Absence of gas within the large bowel (unless recent obstruction).

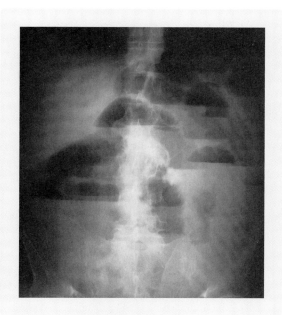

Fig. 21.16 Small bowel obstruction, erect AXR: Evidence of multiple distended small bowel loops containing air-fluid levels, sometimes referred to as a 'stepladder appearance.'

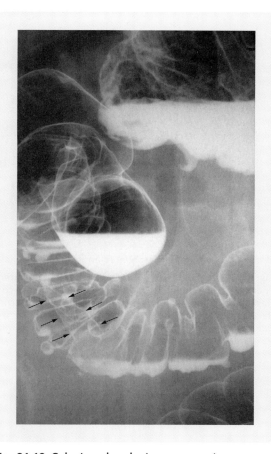

Fig. 21.18 Colonic polyp, barium enema: Appears as a filling defect within bowel mucosa (on air-filled projections polyp may be outlined by contrast) • 50% of polyps occur within 20 cm of the anus • Note subtle polyp (arrows) lying in the sigmoid colon, and coexistent diverticular disease • Associated diverticular disease can mask polyps as these are common coexisting pathologies.

Fig. 21.17 Diverticular disease, barium enema: Smooth outpouchings of bowel (nearly always multiple and varying in size) with contrast within seen as a fluid level.

Fig. 21.19 Familial adenomatous polyposis, barium enema: Bowel 'carpeted' with polyps, seen as small contrast filling defects ● These polyps develop in the second decade of life.

Fig. 21.21 Ulcerative colitis, barium enema: Confluent ulceration of the large bowel ● Loss of haustral markings ● Sometimes described as 'drain pipe' or 'lead pipe' colon.

Fig. 21.20 Colorectal carcinoma, barium enema: Irregular strictured lesion distal to the splenic flexure ● Proximal bowel dilation may herald impending intestinal obstruction ● Classically an 'apple core' appearance with an annular carcinoma ● Loss of normal bowel mucosa ● Shouldering of the lesion.

Fig. 21.23 Sigmoid volvulus, supine AXR: Characteristic 'coffee bean' sign—loops of dilated bowel twisted upon the bowel mesentery • Dilated proximal large bowel loops.

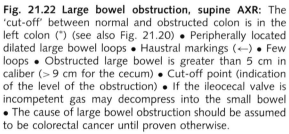

Fig. 21.22 Large bowel obstruction, supine AXR: The 'cut-off' between normal and obstructed colon is in the left colon (*) (see also Fig. 21.20) • Peripherally located dilated large bowel loops • Haustral markings (←) • Few loops • Obstructed large bowel is greater than 5 cm in caliber (> 9 cm for the cecum) • Cut-off point (indication of the level of the obstruction) • If the ileocecal valve is incompetent gas may decompress into the small bowel • The cause of large bowel obstruction should be assumed to be colorectal cancer until proven otherwise.

Fig. 21.24 Ischemic colitis, supine AXR: Thumbprinting due to edema of the bowel mucosa (arrows) • Splenic flexure is the commonest location (due to site of arterial watershed) • Look for other evidence of cardiovascular disease on clinical examination.

Fig. 21.25 Toxic megacolon, thumbprinting on AXR: Dilated large bowel loops with preponderance for transverse colon • Thumbprinting of the bowel mucosa • Find this fast, as it is a cause of bowel perforation and with a high mortality.

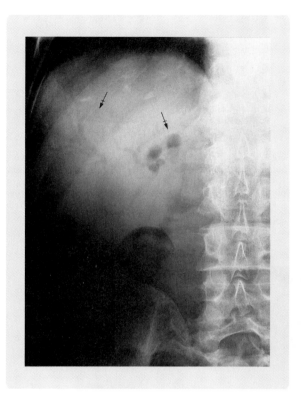

Fig. 22.1 Biliary air, abdominal x-ray (AXR): Tree-like branching pattern (barred arrows) of gas within the liver shadow ● Differential diagnosis—air in portal vein—but portal air tends to be more peripheral.

Fig. 22.2 Cholangiocarcinoma, cholangiogram: Dilated intrahepatic biliary tree (barred arrows) ● Widened biliary radicles ● Look for filling defects within the biliary tree (*) ● Look for continuity of the common bile duct and duodenum.

Fig. 22.3 Gas in biliary tree, CT abdomen: 'Tree-branching' pattern within the liver (barred arrows) • Look for absence of gallbladder or other biliary intervention • Look for biliary stent. (IVC, inferior vena cava; LLL, left lobe liver; LRV, left renal vein; P, pancreas; RLL, right lobe liver; SMA, superior mesenteric artery; ST, stomach; VB, vertebral body.)

Fig. 22.4 Pseudocyst of pancreas, CT abdomen: Typically located in the lesser sac between the stomach and pancreas (see Fig. 22.5). (AO, aorta; LC, left crus of diaphragm; LK, left kidney; LLL, left lobe liver; PC, pseudocyst; RC, right crus of diaphragm; RLL, right lobe liver; SP, spleen.)

Fig. 22.5 Pancreatitis, CT abdomen: Normal pancreatic head/uncinate process (P) enhances normally • Necrotic and inflamed pancreatic body and tail are of lower attenuation (*) • Note inflamed left anterior pararenal plane (barred arrows) characteristic in pancreatitis • Gallstone (arrow) also seen within the gallbladder. (AO, aorta; IVC, inferior vena cava; LK, left kidney; LLL, left lobe liver; RK, right kidney; RLL, right lobe liver.)

Fig. 22.6 Chronic pancreatitis, x-ray: Speckled calcification (arrows) traversing the upper abdomen • Location consistent with the head and body of the pancreas • Look for associated evidence of splenomegaly in portal hypertension.

a

b

Fig. 22.7 (a) Carcinoma (*) of the head of pancreas, CT abdomen: Enlargement of pancreatic head (max. diameter 3 cm normally) • Evidence of distal enlargement of duct and gland atrophy • Absence of fat planes between mesenteric vessels and the pancreas • Metastatic disease, particularly liver, adenopathy. (AO, aorta; D2, second part of duodenum; LK, left kidney; RK, right kidney.) (b) Left renal carcinoma (←). Note left para-aortic lymphadenopathy (*).

133

Fig. 22.8 Common bile duct (CBD), ultrasound: CBD—diameter approximately 6 mm (upper limit of normal) • If enlarged, look for evidence of intrahepatic duct dilatation or failure to taper normally at the lower end • Look for filling defects. (Barred arrow = calculus.)

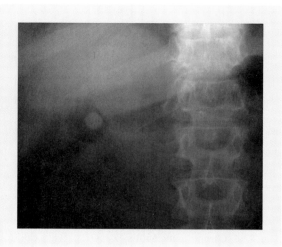

Fig. 22.10 Gallstones, AXR: Laminated calculus identified in the right upper quadrant • Approximately 10–20% gallstones are radiopaque and visible on abdominal radiograph.

Fig. 22.9 Bile duct stones, ERCP: Multiple filling defects (gallstones, barred arrows) within the bile duct • Gallstones also in gallbladder (GB) • Postural imaging may be required to differentiate between calculus and air.

Fig. 22.11 Porcelain gallbladder, AXR: Porcelain bladder calcification of wall of gallbladder • Association with malignancy 20% • Ultrasound may be indicated to exclude calculus.

Fig. 22.12 Operative cholangiogram: Bile duct calculi (barred arrows) • Look for free flow into the duodenum. (CBD, common bile duct; D2, second part of duodenum; D3, third part of duodenum; SS, surgical swab.)

Fig. 22.13 Operative percutaneous transhepatic cholangiogram.

135

Fig. 22.14 Stone in bile duct (arrows), T-tube cholangiogram.

Fig. 22.15 Hepatic metastases, PET-CT scan (Courtesy of Dr J.C. Clarke): Top left: CT scan with metastases in the left lobe • Top right: PET scan showing FDG uptake in the lesion (arrows) • Bottom left: PET-CT fused image, showing the anatomical position of the metabolically active metastasis.

a

b

Fig. 22.16 Normal intravenous urogram: (a) Before contrast administration ('control film') and (b) during examination, with kidneys and ureters visible.

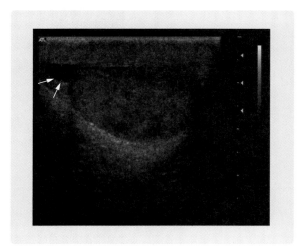

Fig. 22.17 **Ultrasound testes:** epididymal cyst (arrows).

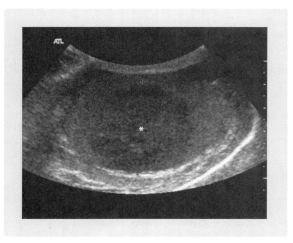

Fig. 22.19 Ultrasound testes: seminoma (*).

Fig. 22.18 **Ultrasound testes:** hydrocele (arrows).

Fig. 22.20 **Ultrasound testes:** varicocele (v). (a) Before, and (b) during Valsalva maneuvre.

137

Fig. 22.21 MRI of stones in the bile duct (arrow).

Fig. 23.1 Pelvic x-ray with sclerotic metastatic bone deposits: These may be bright (sclerotic) or dark (lucent) • Loss of trabecular pattern • Does not begin at a bone end (unlike Paget's disease) • Patient may have known history of primary tumor (in this case prostatic carcinoma).

Fig. 23.3 Fracture of the shaft of the humerus: Loss of normal alignment • Fracture line visible (arrows) • Association with shaft fracture: radial nerve • Association with neck fracture: axillary nerve.

Fig. 23.2 Scaphoid fracture: Lucent line through waist of scaphoid (arrows) • Association: avascular necrosis of proximal fragment.

Fig. 23.4 Boxer's fracture, 5th metacarpal: Fracture line visible through 5th metacarpal bone.

Fig. 23.5 (a) Normal tibia, (b) Paget's disease: Increased convexity of the tibia • Coarsening of the trabecular pattern • Association: sarcoma.

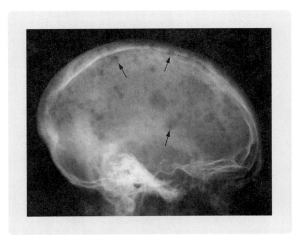

Fig. 23.6 Salt and pepper skull: Multiple lucencies present within the calvarium • Differential diagnosis: (1.) multiple myeloma (2.) hyperparathyroidism.

Fig. 23.8 Rickets: Convexity of both legs • Fraying, splaying and cupping at the epiphysis.

Fig. 23.7 Dynamic hip screw: Internal fixation device with screw through the femoral head and neck and secured to the femoral shaft with screws • Indication: extracapsular fracture with intact blood supply to femoral head.

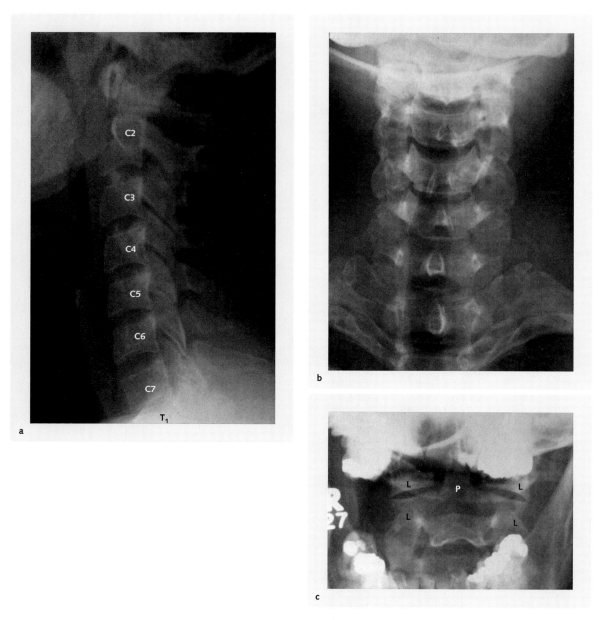

Fig. 23.9 Normal cervical spine x-rays: (a) Lateral; (b) anterior; (c) PEG views; P, odontoid peg ● Confirm all 7 cervical vertebrae and T_1 are visible ● Alignment of vertebrae maintained ● Confirm on PEG view that the lateral masses of C_1 and C_2 (L) line up.

Fig. 23.10 Odontoid peg and teardrop fracture: Etiology is hyperextension ● Both injuries unstable ● Other association of extension teardrop fracture is hangman's fracture.

Fig. 23.11 (a) Osteoblastic L2 and (b) osteolytic L3 vertebrae metastases: Dense bone (arrows (a)) • Most likely underlying cause is prostate or breast cancer or lymphoma • Osteolytic: lucent dark area in bone (arrows (b)) • Absent left pedicle (P) at L3, classic appearance of an 'eye winking.'

a

Fig. 23.13 Gout: Asymmetric involvement of joints • Punched-out erosions away from the joint margin (→ arrows) • Soft tissue swelling (→ arrows).

b

Fig. 23.12 Ankylosing spondylitis: (a) Bamboo spine with (b) sacroiliitis (arrows). Flowing syndesmophytes • Preservation of disc spaces • Multiple contiguous levels affected • Association: pseudofracture • Calcification of anterior spinous ligament (→).

Fig. 23.14 Compression fracture of L2 (a) lateral spine x-ray, (b) T1, and (c) T2 weighted MRI scan: Loss of height in the vertebral body with wedging anteriorly • Decreased T1 and increased T2 signal • Posterior bulging against conus • Look for similar signal change at other levels • Clues to metastatic etiology: normal bone density, other levels affected, known primary tumor, minimal trauma.

Fig. 23.15 Knees with osteoarthritis: Loss of joint space (arrows) • Osteophytic reaction • Sclerotic bone • Subchondral cysts.

Fig. 23.16 Arachnodactyly in Marfan's syndrome: Elongated slender metacarpals • Metacarpal index greater than 8.4.

Fig. 23.17 Psoriatic arthropathy of the foot: Joint space narrowing with associated erosions centered at the MP and IP joint levels • History of psoriasis and overt skin changes.

a

b

Fig. 23.18 Tc99m-MDP isotope bone scan demonstrating multiple metastases (a, b): Images acquired at 2–3 hours following injection • Multiple areas of increased isotope uptake • Asymmetrical distribution • History of known primary.

147

Fig. 23.19 X-ray of the hands in acromegaly: Hands enlarged • Metacarpals and phalanges spade shaped • Prominent tendinous insertions (entheses).

Fig. 23.21 X-ray of rheumatoid arthritis of the hand:
• Joint space narrowing centered on the MCP joints
• Ulnar deviation, swan-necking, boutonnière deformity
• Periarticular ostepenia • Bong erosions.

Fig. 23.20 Tomogram of enlarged pituitary fossa in acromegaly: Widening of the pituitary fossa (*) • Other features include erosion or destruction of the dorsum sella or posterior clinoids • Clinically: bitemporal hemianopia. SS: sphenoid sinus. DS: dorsum sellae.

Fig. 23.22 X-ray of osteosarcoma of the femur (arrows):
• Periosteal reaction • 'Godman's triangle' • 'Sunray spicules.'

Fig. 23.23 X-ray of osteoarthritis of right hip: Loss of joint space on right side • Sclerotic reactive changes • Peripheral osteophytes • Subchondral cysts.

Fig. 23.24 Lateral x-ray—degenerative changes in lumbar spine: Disc space narrowing at the lower lumbar levels (→ arrows) • Osteophytic changes are present at the margins of the vertebral bodies • Gaseous degeneration of L5/S1 disc noted (→ arrow) • Incidental aortic calcification noted.

Fig. 24.1 Normal midline sagittal section, MRI scan (T1).

Fig. 24.3 Axial contrast enhanced CT brain glioma: High grade glioma (arrow 1) with surrounding low density edema (arrow 2) • Heterogenous enhancement with central low density (necrosis) is typical of this tumor • Note marked mass effect with midline shift (arrow 3).

Fig. 24.2 Normal axial non-contrast CT scan at the level of the internal capsule.

a

b

Fig. 24.4 Coronal MRI sequence through temporal lobes, (a) T1 inversion recovery and (b) T2 at the same level: Atrophic low signal hippocampus (a) (arrow 1) with prominent choroidal fissure (arrow 2)—typical features of mesial temporal sclerosis • Abnormal hippocampus high signal in (b) (arrow).

Fig. 24.5 Cerebral angiogram, lateral view, left common carotid artery caroticocavernous sinus fistula: Direct caroticocavernous sinus fistula • There is simultaneous filling of cavernous sinus (arrow 1), superior ophthalmic vein (arrow 2), and internal carotid artery (arrow 3) • Note cortical venous filling indicating high risk of brain hemorrhage without treatment (arrow 4).

Fig. 24.6 Axial non-contrast CT brain: Lack of differentiation between gray and white matter structures, typical of global hypoxic ischemic injury.

Fig. 24.8 Axial non-contrast CT brain: Large acute sub-dural hematoma (SDH) over right frontal and parietal lobes (arrow) ● Crescentic shape is typical of SDH ● Note smaller contralateral SDH (→ arrow).

Fig. 24.9 Axial CT skull base fracture of sphenoid sinus (imaged on bone windows): Sphenoid sinuses opacified with blood (arrow 1) ● Fracture in lateral wall left sphenoid sinus involving adjacent carotid canal (arrow 2).

Fig. 24.7 Cerebral angiogram, intracerebral aneurysm (a) frontal view, right internal carotid artery, (b) aneurysm obliterated by coils (arrow), (c) same but unsubtracted image: Aneurysm in (a) arising at posterior communicating artery origin (arrow 1) ● Note rupture bleb (arrow 2) ● Coils in (b) and (c) clearly seen within the aneurysm (arrows).

153

Fig. 24.11 Large acute extradural hematoma (arrow 1), axial CT: The biconvex shape is typical • Note marked mass effect with midline shift (arrow 2) and effacement of lateral ventricle (arrow 3).

Fig. 24.10 Axial non-contrast CT brain: contusional hemorrhage and diffuse axonal injury (a) Contusional hemorrhage, medial left temporal lobe (arrow 1); brain stem hemorrhage involving midbrain (arrow 2). (b) Diffuse axonal injury; punctate hemorrhage at interface between left thalamus (grey matter) and internal capsule (white matter).

Fig. 24.12 Sagittal (a, b) and axial (c) T2 flair MRI of brain, and (d) T2 MRI of cervical spine demyelination: Nodular foci typical of demyelination seen as bright areas in the corpus callosum (arrow 1 in (a)) and periventricular white matter (arrow 2 in (b) and 3 in (c)) ● Demyelinating plaque posterior upper cervical cord (arrow 4 in (d)).

Fig. 24.13 Axial non-contrast CT brain with diffuse subarachnoid hemorrhage: Hyperdense acute hemorrhage in Sylvian fissures (arrow 1), basal cisterns (arrow 2) and interhemispheric fissure (arrow 3).

Fig. 24.15 Axial contrast enhanced CT brain: Choroid plexus papilloma within right lateral ventricle (arrow 1)
• Note associated hydrocephalus (arrow 2).

Fig. 24.14 CT angiogram: Aneurysm arising from anterior communicating artery (arrow 1).

Fig. 24.17 Axial non-contrast CT brain cerebral thrombosis: Dense middle cerebral artery (arrow) due to acute thrombosis.

Fig. 24.16 Axial (a) and sagittal (b) T$_2$ weighted MRI of ependymoma in 4th ventricle: Bright on T2 MRI (arrow 1 in (a)) with patchy enhancement centrally (arrow 3 in (b))
• Note dilated temporal horns due to hydrocephalus (arrow 2 in (a)).

Fig. 24.19 Axial non-contrast CT brain intracranial hematoma. Large acute intracerebral hematoma (arrow 1) with intraventricular extension (arrow 2) and midline shift (arrow 3).

Fig. 24.18 (a) Axial non-contrast CT brain, (b) Non-contrast sagittal T1 MRI brain colloid cyst: (a) Hyperdense colloid cyst in base of septum pellucidum (arrow 1); note hydrocephalus (arrow 2). (b) Colloid cyst is seen as hyperintense (bright) mass (arrow).

a

c

Fig. 24.20 Meningioma with adjacent edema, (a) axial enhanced CT brain, (b) axial T2 and (c) contrast enhanced T1 MRI: Meningioma (*) better demonstrated on MRI, axial T2 (b) and contrast enhanced axial T1 (c) • Note characteristic enhancing dural tail in (arrow in c).

b

Fig. 24.21 MRI scan: acoustic neuroma (arrows).

Fig. 24.23 Axial T$_2$ weighted MRI: pleomorphic adenoma
● Well circumscribed mass in the right parotid gland (arrows).

Fig. 24.22 Ultrasound scan: thyroid nodule. Solid mass (M) with a fluid center (c).

Fig. 24.24 Parotid gland MRI with Sjögren's syndrome. Axial T$_2$ weighted MRI: Sjögren's syndrome ● Small cysts within the right parotid gland (arrows) ● Association with Non-Hodgkins' lymphoma.

Fig. 24.25 Bilateral carotid body tumors on neck enhanced CT scan: Markedly enhancing masses (M) are noted bilaterally between the splayed internal carotid artery (ICA) and the external carotid artery (ECA).

a

b

c

Fig. 24.26 MRI of a left cheek with lipoma, (a) axial T1 weighted, (b) axial T2 weighted, (c) axial fat suppressed: Lipoma (*) has normal characteristics of fat—high signal on T1 and T2 sequences and completely dark on fat suppression sequences.

161

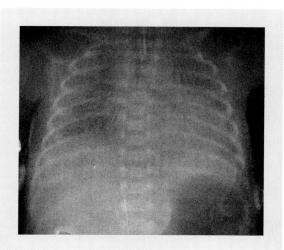

Fig. 25.1 Surfactant deficiency, CXR: Also known as respiratory distress syndrome or hyaline membrane disease • Affects premature infants less than 36 weeks gestational age • Non-compliant lungs are hypoinflated on the CXR • Collapsed alveoli combined with interstitial and alveolar edema lead to bilateral lung opacities • Air bronchograms may be present • Can be complicated by pulmonary hemorrhage or air leaks.

Fig. 25.2 Congenital diaphragmatic hernia, CXR: Most commonly Bochdalek hernias through the left, posterior pleuroperitoneal foramen • Usually diagnosed by antenatal sonography • Prognosis relates to the degree of pulmonary hypoplasia • Initially the CXR shows an opaque hemithorax due to fluid-filled loops of bowel that aerate with time • There is contralateral cardiomediastinal shift • The course of an orogastric tube will confirm if the stomach is lying in the thorax • BochdaLek hernias lie at the Back of the chest, are Big, diagnosed in Babies and lie on the Left side.

163

Fig. 25.3 Necrotizing enterocolitis (NEC), AXR: Primarily affects premature infants • Risk factors include sepsis, umbilical cannulation, hypoxia, and maternal cocaine abuse • Initially, the abdominal x-ray (AXR) is non-specific with diffuse gaseous distension of small and large bowel loops • Disease progression leads to fixed dilatation of one or more loops of bowel, mucosal edema, pneumatosis intestinalis (intramural gas), portal venous gas, and frank perforation • Late complications of NEC include strictures, abscesses, enteric fistulae, malabsorption, and short bowel syndrome following surgical resection.

Fig. 25.4 Duodenal atresia, AXR: Shows the 'double bubble' of the gas-filled stomach and duodenal cap • 80% are distal to the ampulla of Vater • One-third of patients have Down's syndrome • May be diagnosed antenatally • Maternal polyhydramnios and prematurity are common • Neonatal duodenal obstruction may also be due to a duodenal stenosis or web, annular pancreas, or small bowel malrotation and volvulus—all require surgical management.

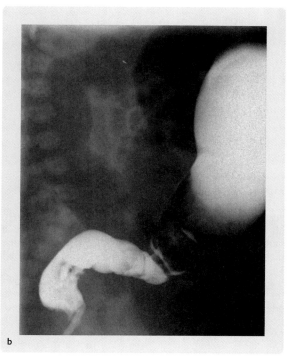

Fig. 25.5 (a) Low bowel obstruction, AXR; (b) Hirschsprung's disease, barium enema: Functional low bowel obstruction due to failure of caudad migration of neuroblasts in developing bowel ● In 75% of cases the point of neuronal arrest is in the rectosigmoid colon ● AXR shows low bowel obstruction, with multiple dilated loops of bowel down to the level of the obstruction, requires barium enema, which may be diagnostic and therapeutic ● Barium enema shows narrow aganglionic (distal) bowel with a funnel-shaped transition zone leading to dilated, normally innervated (more proximal) bowel ● Irregular muscular contractions may be seen in the denervated rectum ● In rectosigmoid Hirschsprung's disease, the sigmoid is more dilated than the rectum (reversal of the normal rectosigmoid ratio) ● Complications of Hirschsprung's disease include bowel perforation and enterocolitis.

Fig. 25.6 Developmental dysplasia of the hip (DDH), ultrasound: Risk factors include breech delivery, positive family history of DDH, abnormal ligamentous laxity, maternal oligohydramnios, and being a female infant • Ultrasound is the imaging method of choice up to 6 months of age • Coronal view with flexed hip shows the iliac bone as a straight vertical line (IB) • The lateral edge of the bony acetabular roof should be sharply angulated—it is rounded or flattened in dysplastic hips (as in this case) • The unossified femoral head (H) should be half to two-thirds covered by the acetabular roof • A dislocated femoral head is displaced superolaterally and posteriorly. (IB: innominate bone. BAR: bony acetabular roof. H: femoral head. CC: cartilage cap.)

Fig. 25.7 Atrioventricular septal defect (AVSD) (also referred to as an AV canal or endocardial cushion defect): Complete AVSD lesion has four components—ASD, VSD, cleft mitral valve, and cleft tricuspid valve (leading to mitral and tricuspid regurgitation, respectively) • CXR shows cardiac enlargement, especially of the atria • Main pulmonary trunk is prominent and there is shunt vascularity • Pulmonary edema may be superimposed • Shunt vascularity means both the pulmonary arteries (arrows) and veins are enlarged due to increase in volume of blood flowing through the pulmonary circulation • Shunt vascularity is synonymous with pulmonary plethora • Echocardiogram will confirm the diagnosis, angiography may also be required • Child with a left-to-right shunt is acyanotic—spotting this is key to formulating the differential diagnosis on CXR of patients with congenital heart disease • Other types of left-to-right shunt include ASD, VSD, PDA, AP window, PAPVD, coronary artery to right atrial fistula and anomalous origin of the left coronary artery when it arises from one of the pulmonary arteries.

166

Fig. 25.8 Fallot's tetralogy: Four components to the tetra-logy—a large VSD with an overriding, anteriorly displaced aorta, pulmonary outflow tract obstruction, and conse-quent right ventricular hypertrophy • Right-sided aortic arch is seen in 25% of patients • CXR shows a 'boot-shaped' heart (coeur en sabot), the heart is moderately enlarged with an upturned apex • The main pulmonary artery segment is concave and the ascending aorta is dilated • The lungs are oligemic due to right-to-left shunt-ing of blood • Echocardiography, angiography and MRI are complementary imaging techniques that may be required.

Fig. 25.9 Small bowel malrotation and volvulus, barium meal: Malrotation describes any variation in the position of the intestines and is associated with a short base to the small bowel mesentery, which predisposes to midgut vol-vulus (twisting of the bowel and compromising its blood supply) • AXR findings are variable and non-diagnostic, upper GI contrast study is necessary to diagnose • The duodeno-jejunal flexure normally lies to the left of the left pedicles, at the same height as the duodenal cap, lying lower and to the right of midline in malrotation • Volvulus can totally occlude the bowel lumen and cause duodenal obstruction • Classically on an upper GI series, volvulus causes a 'corkscrew' pattern of the jejunum spiralling around the mesenteric vessels • Midgut volvulus is a life-threatening condition and requires emergency surgery after diagnosis.

Fig. 25.10 Hypertrophic pyloric stenosis, ultrasound: More common in first-born males who present between the ages of 4 and 6 weeks • Stomach should be filled with clear fluids before the ultrasound to act as an acoustic window through which to scan • Ultrasound features include a canal length > 15 mm (white crosses) and a pyloric muscle thickness > 2.5 mm (arrows) • Increased gastric peristalsis and failure of the pyloric canal to open may also be observed during real-time scanning • Barium meal examination occasionally required to confirm—shows elongated pyloric canal, with indentation of the gastric antrum and delayed gastric emptying.

Fig. 25.11 Vesico-ureteric reflux (VUR), voiding cystour-ethrography (VCUG): May be detected using conventional VCUG, sonographic cystography, direct isotope cystography, or indirect radionuclide cystography • VUR is graded I–V depending upon the severity, grade II+ reaches renal level • VUR is more common in the lower rather than the upper moiety of a duplex system • The bladder (B) and urethra are also demonstrated in a VCUG. (LCS, left (renal) collecting system; LU, left ureter.)

Fig. 25.13 Non-accidental injury (NAI): Skeletal trauma is most common in children <2 years of age • A skeletal survey *not* a 'babygram' is required • Isotope bone scans are useful if the history is suggestive of NAI and skeletal survey negative • CT defines associated intracranial and intra-abdominal injuries • Bone lesions that are of high specificity for NAI include metaphyseal ('corner' or 'bucket-handle') fractures, posterior rib fractures, scapular fractures, spinous process fractures and sternal fractures • All rib fractures are easier to see when they are healing (callus being visible) • Posterior fractures found just lateral to the costo-vertebral junction and usually associated with episodes of shaking • Bilateral subdural hematomas should be considered due to NAI until proven otherwise • Skeletal survey is required to look for other injuries.

Fig. 25.12 Greenstick fracture of ulna and radius: Children's bones can tolerate more deformation than adult bones • Longitudinal compression of a bone results in plastic deformation and a bowing fracture • Continued force causes a torus (buckle) fracture, where the bone's cortex remains intact • Increasing the force further leads to a greenstick (incomplete) fracture in which there is a breach of the bone cortex on the convex side • Failure to remove the force will eventually lead to a complete fracture of the bone.

Fig. 25.14 Perthes' disease: Avascular necrosis of the capital femoral epiphysis, cause unknown • Is bilateral and asymmetric in 10% of cases • Early x-ray signs include fissure fractures, irregularity, and increase in density of capital femoral epiphysis • Later x-ray changes include loss of height, fragmentation, and sclerosis of the femoral head • Cysts may develop in the femoral neck, which broadens, and the outer portion of the dysplastic femoral head may not be covered by the acetabular roof • Reossification and remodelling of the femoral head occur with time, but deformity often persists • Further imaging with isotope bone scans and MRI is occasionally required to help make the diagnosis • Children with hip pathology may present with thigh or knee pain.

Fig. 25.15 Slipped upper femoral epiphysis (SUFE) (also known as SCFE—slipped capital femoral epiphysis): Represents a Salter Harris type I fracture through the proximal femoral growth plate • Both AP and 'frog-leg' lateral views of the hips are required for diagnosis • The AP view may show osteopenia of the femoral head and neck, widening of the growth plate and blurring of the metaphyseal margins • The frog-leg lateral shows the extent of posterior displacement of the femoral head • Avascular necrosis may complicate severe slips • Bilateral disease is not uncommon.

170

Fig. 25.16 Measurement of biparietal diameter during the second trimester, ultrasound: Transverse section of fetal skull, ultrasound calipers positioned from parietal bone to parietal bone.

Fig. 25.17 Measurement of abdominal circumference, fetal ultrasound: Transverse section at the level of the stomach may be used in the third trimester to assess growth and estimate weight.

Fig. 25.18 Measurement of femur length, fetal ultrasound: Longitudinal view of femur obtained—measurement should correspond with biparietal diameter.

Glossary

AAA	abdominal aortic aneurysm		FL	femur length
ABG	arterial blood gas		FNAC	fine needle aspiration cytology
ABPI	ankle brachial pressure index		FNH	focal nodular hyperplasia
AC	abdominal circumference		FVC	forced vital capacity
AF	atrial fibrillation		GCS	Glasgow Coma Scale
ANA	antinuclear antibody		GERD	gastro-esophageal reflux disease
AP	anteroposterior		GI	gastrointestinal
APKD	adult polycystic kidney disease		Hb	hemoglobin
APN	acute pyelonephritis		HC	head circumference
ARDS	acute respiratory distress syndrome		HCC	hepatocellular carcinoma
ASD	atrial septal defect		HCG	human chorionic gonadotrophin
AV	atrioventricular		HIDA	hepatoiminodiacetic acid
AVM	arteriovenous malformation		HOCM	hypertrophic obstructive cardiomyopathy
AVN	avascular necrosis		HPOA	hypertrophic pulmonary osteoarthropathy
AVSD	atrioventricular septal defect		HRCT	high resolution computed tomography
AXR	abdominal x-ray		HS	heart sound(s)
BMI	body mass index		IBD	inflammatory bowel disease
BPD	biparietal diameter		ICA	internal carotid artery
CABG	coronary artery bypass graft		ICH	intracerebral hematoma; intracranial hemorrhage
CAM	cystic adenomatoid malformation			
CBD	common bile duct		ICP	intracranial pressure
CC	corpus callosum		ICU	intensive care unit
CEA	carcinoembryonic antigen		IIH	idiopathic intracranial hypertension
CF	cystic fibrosis		INR	international normalized ratio
CHF	congestive heart failure		IR	inversion recovery
COPD	chronic obstructive pulmonary disease		IUGR	intrauterine growth retardation
CPPD	calcium pyrophosphate deposition disease		IVC	inferior vena cava
CRC	colorectal carcinoma		IVH	intraventricular hemorrhage
CRL	crown–rump length		IVP	intravenous pyelogram
CRP	C-reactive protein		JVP	jugular venous pressure
CSF	cerebrospinal fluid		LA	left atrium
CSP	cavum septum pellucidum		LFT	liver function test
CT	computed tomography		LMP	last menstrual period
CTA	CT angiography		LMWH	low molecular weight heparin
CVA	cerebrovascular accident		LV	left ventricle
CXR	chest x-ray		LVF	left ventricular failure
DAI	diffuse axonal injury		MAA	macroaggregates of albumin
DCBE	double contrast barium enema		MAG-3	mercaptoacetyltriglycene
DDH	developmental dysplasia of the hip		MCP	metacarpophalangeal [joint]
DEXA	dual energy x-ray absorptiometry		MCV	mean corpuscular volume
DIP	distal interphalangeal [joint]		MDP	methylene diphosphonate
DMARD	disease-modifying anti-rheumatic drug		MIBG	meta-iodo-benzyl-guanidine
DMSA	dimercaptosuccinic acid		MIBI	methoxyisobutyl isonitrile
DSA	digital subtraction angiography		MRA	magnetic resonance angiography
DTPA	diethylene triamine pentacetic acid		MRC	magnetic resonance cholangiography
DVT	deep venous thrombosis		MRCP	magnetic resonance cholangiopancreatography
ECA	external carotid artery		MRI	magnetic resonance imaging
ECG	electrocardiogram		MSAFP	maternal serum alphafetoprotein
ED	effective dose		MVA	motor vehicle accident
EDH	epidural hematoma		NAD	no abnormal defect
ERCP	endoscopic retrograde cholangiopancreatography		NAI	non-accidental injury
			NCCT	non-contrast computed tomography
ESM	ejection systolic murmur		NEC	necrotizing enterocolitis
ESR	erythrocyte sedimentation rate		NG	nasogastric [tube]
EVAR	endovascular repair [of abdominal aortic aneurysms]		NM	nuclear medicine
			NRC	Nuclear Regulatory Commission
FBP	full blood picture		NSAID	non-steroidal anti-inflammatory drug
FDG	fluorodeoxyglucose		NT	nuchal translucency
FEV_1	forced expiratory volume in 1 sec		NTD	neural tube defects

OA	osteoarthritis		SCFE	slipped capital femoral epiphysis
OCP	oral contraceptive pill		SDH	subdural hematoma
PA	posteroanterior		SLE	systemic lupus erythematosus
PAPVD	partial anomalous pulmonary venous drainage		SMA	superior mesenteric artery
PCA	percutaneous coronary angioplasty		SOB	shortness of breath
PCom	posterior communicating [artery]		SPECT	single photon emission computed tomography
PDA	patent ductus arteriosus		STIR	short tau inversion-recovery
PE	pulmonary embolus		TAS	transabdominal scan
PEFR	peak expiratory flow rate		TB	tuberculosis
PET	positron emission tomography		TEE	transesophageal echocardiography
PFT	pulmonary function test		TFT	thyroid function test
PIP	proximal interphalangeal [joint]		THR	total hip replacement
PPI	proton pump inhibitor		TIA	transient ischemic attack
PR	per rectum		TTE	transthoracic echocardiography
PTC	percutaneous transhepatic cholangiography		TVUS	transvaginal ultrasound scan
RA	rheumatoid arthritis; right atrium		U&E	urea and electrolytes
RBBB	right bundle branch block		UC	ulcerative colitis
RF	radiofrequency; rheumatoid factor		USS	ultrasound scan
RI	resistive index		UTI	urinary tract infection
RIP	rotation, inspiration, penetration		VCUG	voiding cystourethrogram
RUQ	right upper quadrant		VQ scan	ventilation–perfusion scan
RV	right ventricle		VSD	ventricular septal defect
SAH	subarachnoid hemorrhage		VUR	vesico-ureteric reflux
SB	spina bifida		WBC	white blood count

Index

A

IV gadolinium, 72
abdominal X-ray (AXR), 25
   abdominal aortic aneurysm, 23
   abdominal/pelvic abscess, 24
   aortic stent placement, 115
   appendicitis, 21
   biliary air, 131
   biliary colic, 21–2
   bowel habit, altered, 31, 34, 35
   cholelithiasis, 21–2
   colorectal cancer, 32–3
   Crohn's disease, 31–2
   diverticulosis, 20
   fibroids (leiomyomata), 24
   gallstones, 134
   intestinal ischemia, 21
   ischemic colitis, 129
   large bowel obstruction, 19, 129
   meconium, delayed passage, 67, 68–9, 70
   pancreatic carcinoma, 29
   pancreatitis, 22
   pediatric radiology, 164–5
   phlebolith, 22
   pneumoperitoneum falciform ligament
      sign, 125
   porcelain gallbladder, 134
   pseudo-obstruction, 20
   rectal bleeding, 31
   renal malignancy, 23
   sigmoid volvulus, 129
   small bowel obstruction, 20, 126–7
   ulcerative colitis, 33
abdominal aortic aneurysm, 23–4, 114
abdominal cyst, fetal, 80
abdominal distension, 91
abdominal imaging, 116, 131–8
abdominal mass, 91
abdominal pain, 19–26
   computed tomography, 19
   gynecological diseases, 24–5
   hepatopancreatobiliary diseases, 21–2
   intestinal causes, 19–21
   radiograph *see* abdominal X-ray
   ultrasound, 19
   urological diseases, 22–3
   vascular diseases, 23–4

abortion
   complete, 77
   incomplete, 77
   missed, 77
   threatened, 77
abscess
   abdominal/pelvic, 24–5
   breast, 18
   Brodie's, 50
   drainage, 90
achalasia, 15–16, 121
   esophageal carcinoma, 15
   esophageal diseases, 15–16
acoustic neuroma, 160
acoustic shadow, 21
acromegaly, 44, 148
adenoid cystic carcinoma, 54
adenolymphoma, 54
adenoma, 53
   hepatic, 28
   pleomorphic, 160
adenomatous polyposis, 128
adnexa, 91
adrenal medullary imaging, 96
agenesis of the corpous callosum, 79
AIDS, 7
air
   computed tomography, 90
   radiograph, 87
air bronchogram, 4
alphafetoprotein, 78, 81, 83
amniocentesis, 81
amniotic fluid, 83
   oligiohydramnios, 80, 81
anaplastic carcinoma, 54
ancephaly, 81
anechoic, 27, 91
anembryonic pregnancy, 77
anemia, pernicious, 50
anencephaly, 78–9, 83
aneurysm, 61
   abdominal, 23–4, 38, 114
   aneurysmal bone cyst, 41
   aortic, 19, 114
   cerebral, 57, 58, 156
   dissection, 3, 114
   femoral artery, 38

175

aneurysm *(Continued)*
   intracerebral, 153
   popliteal, 38
   pseudoaneurysn, 38, 39
   ventricular, 113
angiodysplasia, 31, 33–4
angiography
   carotid, 113
   carotid body tumor (chemodectoma;
      paraganglionoma), 55
   catheter, 4
   digital subtraction (DSA), 115
   renal artery, 115
ankle
   tibiotalar slant, 49
ankylosing spondylitis, 41, 48, 145
ankylosis, 47
anorectal atresia, 68
anorectal malformation, 68
anus
   ectopic, 68
   imperforate, 68
   malformation, 68
aorta, 91
   aneurysm *see* aneurysm
   calcification, 114
   coarctation, 13
   stent placement, 115
aortic dissection, 3, 4, 24, 114
   Stanford type B, 9
appendicitis, 21
arachnodactyly, 146
arterial dissection/occlusion, 60
arthritides, inflammatory, 71
arthropathy
   ankylosing spondylitis, 41, 48, 145
   arthritis mutilans, 48
   calcium pyrophosphate dehydrate (CPPD)
      deposition disease, 49
   dactylitis, 48
   degenerative arthritis, 48
   enteropathic, 41, 48
   gout, 49, 145
   hemarthrosis, 49
   hemochromatosis, 50
   hypertrophic pulmonary osteoarthropathy
      (HPOA), 50
   monoarthritis, 48
   oligoarthritis, 48
   osteoarthritis *see* osteoarthritis

arthropathy *(Continued)*
   psoriatic, 41, 47–8, 148
   Reiter's syndrome, 41, 48
   rheumatoid *see* rheumatoid arthritis
   septic arthritis, 49, 71
   seronegative arthritis, 41, 47–8
ascites, 16
aspiration
   fine needle aspiration cytology (FNAC),
      53, 55, 56
   joint, 49
   pneumonia, 7
   transient synovitis of the hip, 71
atlantoaxial joint
   rheumatoid arthritis, 47
atrial enlargement, 114
atrial septal defect, 113
atrioventricular septal defect (AVSD), 166
avascular necrosis (AVN), 75

B
back pain, 41–5
   acromegaly, 44
   ankylosing spondylitis, 41, 145
   bamboo spine, 41, 145
   benign tumors, 41–2
   chordoma, 42
   disc disease, 41, 45
   discitis, 73
   enteropathic arthropathy, 41
   hyperparathyroidism, 44
   inflammatory diseases, 41
   malignant tumors, 42
   metabolic bone disease, 42–4
   myeloma, 42
   neoplastic spinal disease, 41–2
   osteomalacia, 44
   osteoporosis, 42–3
   Paget's disease, 44
   plasmacytoma, 42
   primary bone tumors, 41–2
   psoriatic arthropathy, 41
   Reiter's syndrome, 41
   rickets, 44
   secondary bone tumors, 42
   seronegative arthropathy, 41
bacteriuria, 63
bamboo spine, 41, 145
banana sign, 79
barium enema

barium enema *(Continued)*
    colonic polyp, 127 barium enema
    colorectal carcinoma, 128
    diverticular disease, 127
    familial adenomatous polyposis, 128
    Hirschsprung's disease, 165
    ulcerative colitis, 128
barium meal
    gastric carcinoma, 125
    malrotation, 167
barium swallow, 34, 89
    achalasia, 16, 121
    bowel habit, altered, 34
    candidiasis, 122
    celiac disease, 32
    corrosive stricture, 123
    Crohn's disease, 31, 32
    dysphagia, 15–16, 17
    esophageal carcinoma, 16, 124
    esophageal corrosive stricture, 16
    esophageal varices, 123
    esophageal web, 15, 122
    large bowel obstruction, 19
    pharyngeal pouch, 15, 55, 124
    sceroderma, 32
    small bowel obstruction, 20
    ulcerative colitis, 33
Barlow test, 71
Barrett's esophagus, 16
biliary imaging, 96, 134–5
    bile duct stricture, 29
    biliary air, 131
    calculi, 27, 88
    cholangiocarcinoma, 28
    colic, 21–2
    gallstones, 21–2, 27, 134, 136,
        138
biliary tree, 91, 92
    gas, 132
biparietal diameter (BPD), 78
bladder, 64, 91
    outlet obstruction, 64
Bochdalek hernia, 163
bone
    computed tomography, 90
    fractures, 139
    nuclear medical imaging, 95
    radiograph, 87, 89
    radioisotope scan, 95, 147
    ultrasound, 91

bone density reduction, calculation, 42
bone tumors
    benign, 41–2
    malignant, 42
    secondary, 42
boutonnière deformity, 47
bowel
    bowel habit, altered, 31–5
    bowel lumen polyp, 20
    colonic polyp, 127
    denervated, 69
    displacement, 88
    diverticular disease, 31, 32, 127
    familial adenomatous polyposis, 128
    ganglionated, 69
    gas pattern, 88
    large *see* large bowel
    meconium, delayed passage, 67–70
    neonatal high bowel obstruction, 69
    neonatal low bowel obstruction,
        68–9, 165
    small *see* small bowel
brain hemorrhage, 154, 156
branchial cyst, 55
breast
    abscess, 118
    breast mass, 13, 14
    carcinoma, 117–19
    mammography, 13–14,
        116–19
    screening, 13–14
Brodie's abscess, 50
bronchiectasis, 106
bronchoalveolar carcinoma, 8
bronchoalveolar lymphoma, 8
bronchogenic carcinoma, 3
Budd-Chiari syndrome, 91

C
calcium pyrophosphate dehydrate (CPPD)
    deposition disease, 49
Candida, 64
candidiasis, 122
caput medusae, 16
carcinoma
    adenoid cystic, 54
    breast, 117–19
    colorectal, 31, 128
    esophageal, 16, 17, 124
    gastric, 125

carcinoma *(Continued)*
   lung, 109
   mucoepidermoid, 54
   parotid, 54
   thyroid mass, 53–4
cardiac failure, 114
cardiac imaging, 91–2, 95
cardiomegaly, 3, 114
cardiovascular disorders, 3–4
caroticocavernous fistula, 60, 152
carotid body tumor, 55, 161
catheter angiography, 57
cecal volvulus, 20
celiac disease, 32
cerebral thrombosis, 157
cerebrospinal fluid (CSF)
   overproduction, 57
   pathway, obstruction, 57
cerebrovascular accident (CBA), 58
Ceretec, 96
cervix, 91
chemodectoma, 55
chest X-ray (CXR)
   achalasia, 15, 121
   aortic coarctation, 13
   apical, 88
   apical carcinoma, 109
   apical tuberculosis, 106
   atrial enlargement, 114
   atrial septal defect, 113
   bilateral pulmonary fibrosis, 107
   bronchiectasis, 106
   cardiac failure, 114
   cavitating lung, 109
   chest pain, dyspnea or hemoptysis, 3–4, 9–10
   collapsed lung, 112
   dysphagia, 15, 17
   emphysema, 105
   esophageal carcinoma, 16
   frontal, 87
   hiatus hernia, 15, 16, 125
   hilar mass, 109, 116
   lateral, 87
   lower lobe consolidation, 107
   mastectomy, 116
   mesothelioma, 110
   miliary tuberculosis, 112
   nipple markers, 104
   nipple shadows, 104
   pectus excavatum, 112
   pediatric radiology, 163

chest X-ray (CXR) *(Continued)*
   pericardial effusion, 116
   pleural effusion, 111
   pneumonia, 4, 108
   pneumoperitonem, 124–5
   pneumothorax, 7–8, 108
   pulmonary embolus, 7
   pulmonary metastases, 111
   renal malignancy, 23
   sarcoidosis, 110
   surfactant deficiency, 163
   thoracic malignancy, 8
   thyroid mass, 15
   ventricular aneurysm, 113
chest pain, 3–11, 87
chest radiograph (CXR), 103–4
Chilaiditi's sign, 21
chocolate cyst, 24
cholangiocarcinoma, 131
   extrahepatic, 29
   hilar (Klatskin tumor), 28–9
   peripheral, 28
cholangiogram, 131, 135–6
cholecystectomy, history of, 21
choledochal cyst, fetal, 80
cholelithiasis
   abdominal X-ray, 21–2
   computed tomography, 22
   endoscopic retrograde
      cholangiopancreatography, 22
   magnetic resonance cholangiography, 22
   magnetic resonance imaging, 22
chondrocalcinosis, 49, 50
chordoma, 42
chrondrolysis
   slipped capital femoral epiphysis (SCFE), 73
chronic obstructive pulmonary disease
      (COPD), 9–10
cirrhosis, 27, 28
   esophageal varices, 16
cleft palate, 81
CLUBBING, 50
coffee-bean sign, 20
colon *see* large bowel
colonic atresia, 68
colonic polyp, 127
colonic stenosis, 68
colonography, 31, 32–3
colonoscopy, 34
colorectal cancer, 32–3, 129
   Gardner's syndrome, 32

colorectal carcinoma, 31, 128
common bile duct, 134
computed tomography (CT), 87, 90
    abdomen, 116, 132–3
    abdominal aortic aneurysm, 23–4
    abdominal pain, 19, 25
    abdominal/pelvic abscess, 25
    aortic dissection, 4, 24, 114
    appendicitis, 21
    attenuation value, 90
    bilateral pulmonary fibrosis, 107
    bile duct stricture, 29
    bone density reduction, 42
    bowel habit, altered, 31, 34–5
    branchial cyst, 55
    bronchiectasis, 106
    chest pain, dyspnea or hemoptysis, 3, 9, 10,
        11, 104, 105
    cholangiocarcinoma, 28–9
    cholelithiasis, 22
    chordoma, 42
    cirrhosis, 27
    colonography, 31, 32–3
    colorectal cancer, 32–3
    contrast enhanced, 23, 110
    cranial, 57
    CT drainage, 35
    cystic hygroma, 55
    dysphagia, 15, 17
    ectropic/undescended testicle, 38
    emphysema, 105
    esophageal carcinoma, 16
    esophageal varices, 16
    focal neurological deficit, 58
    head and neck, 151–4, 156–9, 161
    helical, 23–4
    hemangioma, 27
    hematoma, 153, 154
    hepatocellular carcinoma, 28
    hips, 74
    Hounsfield units (HU), 90
    hydatid disease, 28
    inguinal hernia, 38
    intestinal ischemia, 21
    jaundice, 27
    large bowel obstruction, 19
    laryngocele, 55
    liver metastases, 28
    lung carcinoma, 109
    lymphangioma, 55
    multidetector (multislice), 4, 7, 23–4, 90

computed tomography (Continued)
    neck mass, 53
    neurological symptoms, 57–61
    osteoporosis, 42
    pancreatic carcinoma, 29–30, 133
    pancreatitis, 22, 132–3
    parotid (pleomorphic) adenoma, 54
    PET-CT, 94, 136
    pixels, 90
    pneumoperitonem, 21
    pulmonary angiographic algorithm, 11
    pulmonary angiography, 3
    pulmonary embolus, 7, 110
    radiation dose, 19, 87, 90
    rectal bleeding, 31
    renal colic, 22
    renal malignancy, 23
    seizures, 59
    single photon emission computed tomography
        (SPECT), 93
    small bowel obstruction, 20
    subarachnoid hemorrhage, 57
    thyroglossal (duct) cyst, 54
    thyroid mass, 15
    traumatic brain injury, 59–60
    urinary tract infection, 64
    voxel, 90
    Warthin's tumor (adenolymphoma), 54
computed tomography angiography
        (CTA), 57, 156
congenital cyctic adenomatoid malformation
        (CCAM), 79
corpous callosum, agenesis, 79
corrosive stricture, 123
Crohn's disease, 31, 41, 48, 126
crown-rump length (CRL)
        measurement, 77
cup and pencil deformity, 48
cystic fibrosis, 67
cystic hygroma, 55

D

dactylitis, 48
Dandy-Walker syndrome, 79
Dawson's fingers, 58
development dysplasia of the hip (DDH),
        71, 166
diethylene triamine pentacetic acid (DTPA),
        23, 95
diffuse axonal injury (DAI), 60
digital rectal examination (DRE), 31

digital subtraction angiography (DSA), 115
dimercaptosuccinic acid (DMSA), 23, 63, 65, 95
diplopia, 58
disc disease, 41
discitis, 73
distal interphalangeal (DIP) joint, 48
diverticular disease, 31, 32, 127
diverticulosis, 20
diverticulum, perforated, 21
double contract barium enema (DCBE), 32
double contrast enema, 31
Douglas, pouch of, 24
Down's syndrome, 67, 78
dual energy X-ray absorptiometry
    (DEXA), 43–4
duodenal atresia, fetal, 80, 164
duodenal ulcer, 19, 21
dural sinus laceration/occlusion, 60
dysphagia, 15–17
dysphasia
  focal neurological deficit, 58
dysplasia
  hip, 73
dyspnea, 3–11, 87

E
echocardiography, 91, 116
echopoor mass, 83
ectopic pregnancy, 24, 78
electroencephalogram (EEG), 59
emphysema, 105
empty cecum sign, 20
encephalocele, 79
endocardial cushion defect, 166
endoluminal ultrasound, 15
endometrioma, 24
endometriosis, 24
endoscopic retrograde cholangiopancreatography
    (ERCP)
  bile duct stones, 134
  bile duct stricture, 29
  cholelithiasis, 22
  extrahepatic, 29
  jaundice, 27
  pancreatic carcinoma, 30
endoscopy
  esophageal candidiasis, 15
  pneumoperitonem, 21
endovascular occlusion, 61
enteroclysis, 32
enterocolitis, 67

enteropathic arthropathy, 41
ependymoma, 157
epididymal cyst, 37, 137
epilepsy, 58–9
esophageal atresia, fetal, 80
esophageal candidiasis, 15
esophageal carcinoma, 16, 17, 124
esophageal corrosive stricture, 16
esophageal disease, 15–16
esophageal varices, 16, 123
esophageal web, 15, 122

F
falciform ligament sign, 21, 125
Fallot's tetralogy, 167
fat
  computed tomography, 90
  radiograph, 87
  ultrasound, 91
feces, blood in, 31–5
fetal abnormality, 78–80, 82
fetal biometry, 80–1
fetal death, 83
fetal hydrops, 82
fibroadenoma, 116
fibroids, 24, 82
fine needle aspiration cytology (FNAC),
    53, 55, 56
flip-flop pattern, 32
fluorodeoxyglucose (FDG), 33, 94
focal neurological deficit, 57–8
follicular carcinoma, 53–4
foot
  gout, 49
  psoriatic arthropathy, 48, 147
foreign body
  computed tomography, 90
  radiograph, 87, 112, 141
fracture, 139
  compression, 146
  greenstick (incomplete), 169
  hangman's, 143
  non-accidental injury, 169
  odontoid peg and teardrop, 143
  sphenoid sinus, 153
  torus (buckle), 169

G
gallbladder, 91
  porcelain, 134
gallium, 96

gallstones, 21–2, 27, 134, 138
Gardner's syndrome, 32
gas, ultrasound, 91
gastric carcinoma, 125
gastro-esophageal reflux disease (GERD), 16
gastrogaffin, 89
gastrointestinal imaging, 15–16, 89, 97, 121–30
    meconium, delayed passage, 67, 69, 70
gastroschisis, 80
geode, 48
gestational trophoblastic disease, 78
giant cell tumor, 41–2
Glasgow Coma Scale (CGS), 58, 59
glioma, 151
glucose-avid lesion, 8, 94
gout, 49, 145
    chronic tophaceous, 49
groin mass, 37, 38–9
growth hormone, acromegaly, 44
gynecological diseases
    abdominal pain, 24–5
    abdominal/pelvic abscess, 24–5
    ectopic pregnancy, 24
    endometriosis, 24
    fibroids (leiomyomata), 24
    ovarian cyst, torsion, 24
    pelvic inflammatory disease, 25

H
HAG 02, 42
halo sign, 53
hand
    acromegaly, 148
    boxer's fracture, 139
    finger clubbing, 50
    Marfan's syndrome, 146
    osteoarthritis, 47
    psoriatic arthropathy, 48
    rheumatoid arthritis, 47, 50–1, 148
head and neck imaging, 151–61
head trauma, 57, 59–60
headache, 57, 58
heart
    cardiac failure, 114
    cardiac ultrasound, 91–2
    ischemic heart disease, 3
hemangioma, 27–8, 41
hemarthrosis, 49
hematoma, 158
    extradural (ED) ·
    intracere'

hematoma (Continued)
    subdural (SDH), 59–60, 153
hematuria, 19
hemidiaphragm, elevation, 6
hemiparesis, 57–8
hemochromatosis, 50
hemophilia, 49
hemoptysis, 3–11, 87
hemorrhoids, 31, 34
hepatic metastases, 136
hepatitis, 28
    acute, 27
    chronic, 27
hepatobiliary pain, 19
hepatobiliary ultrasound, 91
hepatocellular carcinoma, 28
hepatoma, 16
hepatopancreatobiliary diseases, 21–2
hernia
    Bochdalek, 163
    fetal diaphragmetic, 80, 163
    hiatus see hiatus hernia
    inguinal, 38
    large bowel obstruction, 20
    small bowel obstruction, 20
hiatus hernia, 15, 16, 125
    paraesophageal, 16
    rolling, 16
    sliding, 16
hilar mass, 8, 109, 116
hilum, depression, 6
hip
    computed tomography (CT) scan, 74
    development dysplasia (DDH), 71, 166
    dysplasia, 73
    magnetic resonance imaging (MRI), 74
    osteoarthritis, 47, 149
    pelvic radiography, 73
    Perthes' disease, 72, 170
    rheumatoid arthritis, 47
    slipped capital femoral epiphysis
        (SCFE), 72–3, 74–5
    transient synovitis, 71
    ultrasound, 73
'ppocampal sclerosis, 58
·schsprung's disease, 67, 69, 165
    ›prosencephaly, 79
    ›sfield units (HU), 90
    ı chorionic gonadotrophin (HCG), 78
    s, fracture, 139
    ›embrane disease, 163

Pediatric Radiology

Fig. 25.9 Small bowel malrotation and volvulus, barium meal: Malrotation describes any variation in the position of the intestines and is associated with a short base to the small bowel mesentery, which predisposes to midgut volvulus (twisting of the bowel and compromising its blood supply) • AXR findings are variable and non-diagnostic, upper GI contrast study is necessary to diagnose • The duodeno-jejunal flexure normally lies to the left of the left pedicles, at the same height as the duodenal cap, lying lower and to the right of midline in malrotation • Volvulus can totally occlude the bowel lumen and cause duodenal obstruction • Classically on an upper GI series, volvulus causes a 'corkscrew' pattern of the jejunum spiralling around the mesenteric vessels • Midgut volvulus is a life-threatening condition and requires emergency surgery after diagnosis.

': Four components to the tetra-
n overriding, anteriorly displaced
›w tract obstruction, and conse-
hypertrophy • Right-sided aortic
of patients • CXR shows a 'boot-
er en sabot), the heart is moderately
upturned apex • The main pulmonary
concave and the ascending aorta is
gs are oligemic due to right-to-left shunt-
hocardiography, angiography and MRI are
y imaging techniques that may be required.

hydrocele, 37, 137
hydrocephalus, 57, 156
hydronephrosis, 19, 63
hydrops, fetal, 82
hydrosalpinx, 25
hypaque, 19
hyperechoic, 27, 91
hyperfunctioning nodule, 53
hyperparathyroidism, 22, 44
hyperplasia, fibromuscular, 115
hypertension, 58
hypertrophic pulmonary osteoarthropathy
        (HPOA), 50
hypertrophic pyloric stenosis, 168
hyperuricemia, 49

I
ileal atresia, 67, 70
immunosuppressed patients, 7
indium, 93, 97
infantile polycystic kidney disease, 80
inflammatory bowel disease, 31, 32
inguinal/thigh mass, 38
insulinoma, 97
intercranial pressure (ICP), 57
interventional radiology, 90
intestinal ischemia, 21
intrauterine growth retardation (IUGR), 81, 82
intravenous pyelogram (IVP), 22
intraventricular hemorrhage (IVH), 60
inverted stirrup sign, 55
iodine, 93, 95
ionizing radiation, 19, 87–90
iopamidol, 19, 89
irritable bowel syndrome, 31
ischemic colitis, 21, 129
isotopes, 93–9
    bone scans, 44, 73–4, 147
    thyroid studies, 15

J
jaundice, 27–30, 91
    hepatitis, 27
jejunal atresia, 67
    fetal, 80
joint pain, 47–51
    Brodie's abscess, 50
    calcium pyrophosphate dehydrate (CPPD)
        deposition disease, 49
    gout, 49, 145
    hemochromatosis, 50

joint pain (Continued)
    hemophilia, 49
    hypertrophic pulmonary osteoarthropathy
        (HPOA), 50
    osteoarthritis, 47, 146
    osteomyelitis, 50
    radiograph, 47, 89
    rheumatoid arthritis, 47
    seronegative arthritis, 47–8

K
Kerley B lines, 4, 114
kidney, 91
    congenital dysplastic, 63
    duplex, 63, 64
    horseshoe, 63
    infantile polycystic kidney disease, 80
    multicystic dysplastic, 64
    nuclear medical imaging, 95
    radioisotope scan, 95
    ultrasound, 91
    urinary tract infection, 23, 63–5
Killian's dehiscence, 15, 55, 124
Klatskin tumor, 28–9
knee
    osteoarthritis, 47, 146
    rheumatoid arthritis, 47
krypton, 95

L
large bowel
    angiodysplasia, 33–4
    colonic tuberculosis, 130
    colorectal cancer, 32–3
    diverticular disease, 31, 32
    functionally immature colon, 67
    Gardner's syndrome, 32
    inflammatory bowel disease, 32
    microcolon, 69
    obstruction, 19, 129
    pseudomembranous colitis, 34
    small left colon, 67
    toxic megacolon, 33, 130
    tuberculosis, colonic, 33
    ulcerative colitis, 33, 128
laryngocele, 55
Legg-Calvé-Perthes' disease, 72, 170
leiomyomata, 24
lemon sign, 79
leukemia, 37, 71
lightbulb sign, 28

182

Fig. 25.10 Hypertrophic pyloric stenosis, ultrasound: More common in first-born males who present between the ages of 4 and 6 weeks • Stomach should be filled with clear fluids before the ultrasound to act as an acoustic window through which to scan • Ultrasound features include a canal length > 15 mm (white crosses) and a pyloric muscle thickness > 2.5 mm (arrows) • Increased gastric peristalsis and failure of the pyloric canal to open may also be observed during real-time scanning • Barium meal examination occasionally required to confirm—shows elongated pyloric canal, with indentation of the gastric antrum and delayed gastric emptying.

Fig. 25.11 Vesico-ureteric reflux (VUR), voiding cystourethrography (VCUG): May be detected using VCUG, sonographic cystography, direct isotope phy, or indirect radionuclide cystography • VUR is graded I–V depending upon the severity, grade II+ reflux up to upper level • VUR is more common in the lower rather than the moiety of a duplex system • The bladder, urethra (renal) collecting system; LU, left ureter.) (LU

168

limp, childhood, 71–5
lipoma, 55, 161
liver, 91
    cirrhosis, 27, 28
    focal lesion, 27–8
    focal nodular hyperplasia, 28
    hemangioma, 27–8
    hepatic adenoma, 28
    hepatic cyst, 27
    hepatitis, 27, 28
    hepatocellular carcinoma, 28
    hydatid disease, 28
    metastases, 28
    nuclear medical imaging, 96
loin pain, 19
Looser's zones, 44
lung
    apical chest radiograph, 88
    bilateral pulmonary fibrosis, 107
    carcinoma, 109
    cavitating, 109
    collapsed, 112
    emphysema, 105
    pulmonary angiography, 3
    pulmonary edema, 4, 114
    pulmonary embolus, 3, 7, 94, 104, 110
    pulmonary metastases, 9, 111
    scan see ventilation-perfusion (VQ) scan
    sequestration, fetal, 79
    veiling, 4
lung mass, calcified, 8
lymphadenopathy, 38, 54, 117
lymphangiography, 95
lymphangioma, 55
lymphoma, 37
    celiac disease, 32

M
macroaggregates of albumin (MAA), 94–5
macrosomia, 81, 82
magnetic resonance (MR), 87, 92
magnetic resonance angiography (MRA), 92
magnetic resonance cholangiography (MRC)
    bile duct stricture, 29
    cholelithiasis, 22
    jaundice, 27
    pancreatitis, 22
magnetic resonance cholangiopancreatography
        (MRCP), 92
magnetic resonance imaging (MRI)
    bone tumors, 42

magnetic resonance imaging (MRI) (Continued)
    branchial cyst, 55
    breast mass, 13
    carotid body tumor (chemodectoma;
        paraganglionoma), 55, 161
    cervical spine, 155
    cholangiocarcinoma, 28–9
    cholelithiasis, 22
    chordoma, 42
    colorectal cancer, 33
    cystic hygroma, 55
    Dawson's fingers, 58
    disc disease, 41
    discitis, 73
    ectopic/undescended testicle, 38
    fat suppression sequence, 92
    fibroids (leiomyomata), 24
    focal nodular hyperplasia, 28
    gallstones, 138
    head and neck, 151–2, 155, 157–60
    hemangioma, 27–8
    hepatic adenoma, 28
    hepatic cyst, 27
    hepatocellular carcinoma, 28
    hip and pelvis, 74
    hydatid disease, 28
    inguinal hernia, 38
    inversion recovery (IR) sequence, 92
    lipoma, 55, 161
    liver metastases, 28
    lumbar spine, 45
    lymphangioma, 55
    multiple sclerosis, 58
    neck mass, 53
    neurological symptoms, 57–9
    osteomyelitis, 50
    parotid (pleomorphic) adenoma, 54
    pelvis, 26
    Perthes' disease, 72
    precession, 92
    renal scarring, 64
    sclerosis, 152
    sebaceous cyst, 55
    seizures, 59
    T1 relaxation, 92
    T2 relaxation, 92
    T2 weighted, 146
    thoracic malignancy, 8
    thyroglossal (duct) cyst, 54
    traumatic brain injury, 59–60
    urinary tract infection, 64

magnetic resonance imaging (MRI) *(Continued)*
  Warthin's tumor (adenolymphoma), 54
mammography, 13–14, 116–19
Marfan's syndrome, 146
mastectomy, 116
maternal serum alphafetoprotein (MSAFP),
    78, 81, 83
meconium, delayed passage, 67–70
meconium ileus, 67
meconium plug syndrome, 67
megaBecquerel (MBq), 93
meningioma, 58, 159
mesenteric angiography, 31
mesothelioma, 110
meta-iodo-benzyl-guanidine (MIBG), 96
metacarpophalangeal (MCP) joint, rheumatoid
    arthritis, 47
methotrexate, 51
methoxyisobutyl isonitrile (MIBI), 95
methylene diphosphonate (MDP), 73–4
microcolon, 69
microsencephaly, 79
milliSievert (mSv), 93
molar pregnancy, 78
monoarthritis, 48
moulage sign, 32
mucoepidermoid carcinoma, 54
multiple sclerosis, 58
Mycobacterium tuberculosis, 64
myeloma, 42
myocardial perfusion imaging, 95

N
neck mass, 53–6
  adenoma, 53
  benign mixed tumor of the parotid, 54
  branchial cyst, 55
  carotid body tumor, 55, 161
  chemodectoma, 55
  cystic hygroma, 55
  fine needle aspiration cytology, 53, 55–6
  laryngocele, 55
  lipoma, 55
  lymphadenopathy, 54
  lymphangioma, 55
  paraganglionoma, 55
  parotid carcinoma, 54
  parotid (pleomorphic) adenoma, 54
  pharyngeal pouch, 55
  salivary diseases, 54
  sebaceous cyst, 55

neck mass *(Continued)*
  Sjögren's syndrome, 54, 160
  Sloane-Kettering Level I–VI classification, 53
  thyroglossal (duct) cyst, 54
  thyroid mass, 53–4
  ultrasound, 55–6
  Warthin's tumor (adenolymphoma), 54
necrotizing enterocolitis (NEC), 164
nephrogram, 90
neural tube defects (NTDs), 78–9
neurological symptoms, 57–65, 91
  cerebral aneurysm, 57
  focal neurological deficit, 57–8
  Glasgow Coma Scale, 58, 59
  head and neck imaging, 151–61
  head trauma, 57, 59–60
  headache, 57, 58
  seizures, 58–9
  subarachnoid hemorrhage, 57
Niopam, 19
nipple markers, 87, 104
nipple shadows, 104
non-contrast computed tomography (NCCT)
  hematoma, 59
  intraventricular hemorrhage, 60
non-Hodgkin's lymphoma, 54
nuchal translucency (NT), 78
nuclear medical imaging, 25, 93–9
  adrenal medullary, 96
  biliary imaging, 96
  bone, 95
  cardiac imaging, 95
  chronic infection, 96
  dimercaptosuccinic acid (DMSA), 23, 63, 95
  isotopes, 93
  kidney, 95
  liver, 96
  lymphangiography, 95
  parathyroid, 95
  pertechnetate, 63
  positron emission tomography *see* positron
      emission tomography (PET)
  radiation doses, 97–8
  red cell imaging, 96
  requests, 97
  single photon emission computed tomography
      (SPECT), 93
  spleen, 96
  Tc-labelled MAG-3, 63
  thyroid, 95
  tumor imaging, 97

nuclear medical imaging *(Continued)*
    ventilation-perfusion *see* ventilation-perfusion
        (VQ) scan
    white cell imaging, 96

O
obstetric ultrasound, 77–83
obstructive uropathies, 63
    fetal, 80
octreotide, 25, 97
oligemia, 7
oligiohydramnios, 80, 81
oligoarthritis, 48
omphalocele, 80
organomegaly, 88
orthopedic imaging, 139–50
Ortolani test, 71
osteoarthritis, 47, 48, 149
    hand, 47
    hip, 47
    knee, 47, 146
    primary (polyarticular), 48
    secondary (monoarticular), 48
osteoblastoma, 42, 144
osteodystrophy, renal, 74–5
osteoid
    osteoma, 42
    rickets, 44
    osteolytic metastases, 144
    osteomalacia, 44
    osteomyelitis, 50, 71, 73
    subacute, 50
    osteopenia, 43
    hemophilia, 49
osteophyte, 8
osteoporosis, 42–4
osteosarcoma, 149
ovarian cyst, torsion, 24
ovaries, 91

P
Paget's disease, 44, 140
    lytic, 44
    mixed, 44
    pelvic, 44
    sclerotic, 44
pancreas, 91
    carcinoma, 27, 29–30, 133
    pseudocyst, 132
pancreatitis, 132
    acute, 22

pancreatitis *(Continued)*
    chronic, 22, 133
papillary carcinoma, 53
paraganglionoma, 55
paralytic ileus, 34
parathyroid, 95
parotid
    adenoma, 54
    benign mixed tumor of, 54
    carcinoma, 54
    Sjögren's syndrome, 54, 160
Paterson-Brown Kelly syndrome, 15, 122
PEAR, 41
pectus excavatum, 112
pediatric radiology, 77–83, 163–71
    abortion, threatened, 77
    amniocentesis, 81
    anembryonic, 77
    anencephaly, 78–9, 83
    confirmation of date, 77, 80–1, 82
    confirmation of pregnancy, 77
    congenital cardiac disorders, 79
    congenital thoracic disorders, 79–80
    crown-rump length (CRL), 77
    ectopic, 24, 78
    fetal abnormality, screening for, 78–80
    fetal biometry, 80–1
    fetal death, 81, 83
    fetal distress, 82
    fetal hydrops, 82
    first trimester ultrasound, 77–8
    gastroschisis, 80
    intrauterine growth retardation (IUGR), 81
    large for dates, 81–2
    maternal diabetes, 82
    maternal serum alphafetoprotein (MSAFP),
        78, 81, 83
    molar (gestational trophoblastic disease), 78
    multiple gestation, 78, 81, 82
    omphalocele, 80
    placental abruption, 83
    second trimester ultrasound, 78–81, 171
    small for dates, 81
    third trimester ultrasound, 81–3
    ultrasound, 77–83, 91
    uterine mass, 81, 82
    vaginal bleeding, 82–3
    viable pregnancy, 77
pelvi-ureteric junction obstruction, 63, 64
pelvis
    hemophilic pseudotumor, 49

pelvis *(Continued)*
   magnetic resonance imaging (MRI), 74
   Paget's disease, 44
   pelvic inflammatory disease, 25
   radiograph, 73, 88, 139
   ultrasound, 91
percutaneous transhepatic cholangiography
   (PTC), 27
   extrahepatic, 29
perfusion scan *see* ventilation-perfusion
   (VQ) scan
pericardial effusion, 116
pericardial tamponade, 3
pericarditis, 4
pertechnetate, 63
Perthes' disease, 72, 170
phaeochromocytoma, 96
pharyngeal pouch, 15, 55, 124
phlebolith, 22
pituitary fossa, 148
placenta previa, 82
placental abruption, 83
plasmacytoma, 42
pleomorphic adenoma, 54
pleural effusion, 4, 111
   fetal, 79–80
Plummer-Vinson syndrome, 15, 122
Pneumocystis jiroveci, 108
pneumonia, 4–7
   aspiration, 7
   bronchopneumonia, 4, 7
   cavitating, 4, 7
   Gram-negative, 7
   interstitial, 4, 7
   lobar, 4, 6
   Pneumocystis jiroveci, 108
pneumoperitonem, 21, 88, 124–5
pneumothorax, 3, 7–8, 108
polo-mint sign, 7, 11
polycystic kidney disease, 29
polyhydramnios, 81–2
positron emission tomography (PET), 93–4
   bowel habit, altered, 35
   dysphagia, 17
   esophageal malignancy, 15, 16
   lymphadenopathy, 54
   neck mass, 53
   PET-CT, 94, 136
   thoracic malignancy, 8
   Warthin's tumor (adenolymphoma), 54
posterior fossa tumor, 57

precession, 92
pregnancy *see* pediatric radiology
proximal interphalalangeal (PIP) joint,
   osteoarthritis, 47
pseudoaneurysnm, 38, 39
pseudogout, 49
pseudomembranous colitis, 34
pseudoneuropathy, 49
psoriatic arthropathy, 41, 47–8, 148
psuedofractures
   osteomalacia, 44
pulmonary angiography, 3
pulmonary edema, 4, 114
pulmonary embolus, 3, 7, 94, 104, 110
pulmonary metastases, 9, 111
pyelogram, 90
pyelonephritis, 63, 64
pyosalpinx, 25

R
radiofrequency (RF) pulse, 92
radiograph, 87–90
   abdominal *see* abdominal X-ray
   acromegaly, 44, 148
   ankylosing spondylitis, 145
   back pain, 41–5
   Brodie's abscess, 50
   calcium pyrophosphate dehydrate (CPPD)
      deposition disease, 49, 50
   cervical spine, 88, 142
   chest *see* chest X-ray
   chordoma, 42
   computed tomography *see* computed
      tomography
   development dysplasia of the hip (DDH), 71
   disc disease, 41
   discitis, 73
   dyspnea, 87
   foreign body, 87, 112, 141
   fractures, 139
   gastrointestinal imaging *see* barium swallow
   gout, 145
   hemochromatosis, 50
   joint pain, 47, 89
   laryngocele, 55
   limb X-rays, 89
   lumbar spine, 73, 88
   nipple markers, 87, 104
   osteoarthritis, 149
   osteomalacia, 44
   osteomyelitis, 50, 73

radiograph *(Continued)*
  osteoporosis, 42
  osteosarcoma, 149
  parotid carcinoma, 54
  pelvic, 73, 88, 139
  Perthes' disease, 72
  Reiter's syndrome, 48
  rheumatoid arthritis, 47, 50, 148
  rickets, 44, 141
  scoliosis, 73
  septic arthritis, 71
  slipped capital femoral epiphysis (SCFE), 72–3
  spinal, 88, 142, 150
  thoracic spine, 88
  tissue differentiation, 87
  toddler's fracture, 73
  urography, 89–90
  Warthin's tumor (adenolymphoma), 54
radioisotopes, 93–9
radiolabel led red cell scan, 31
radiopharmeceuticals, 93–9
  quantity (dose), 93
rectal bleeding, 31–5
rectum, malformation, 68
red cell imaging, 96
Reiter's syndrome, 41, 48
renal agenesis, 80, 81
renal calculi, 22, 63, 88, 90
renal colic, 22
renal malignancy, 23
renal metastases, 9
renal osteodystrophy, 74–5
respiratory disorders, 3, 4–9, 103–12
respiratory distress syndrome, 163
rheumatoid arthritis, 47
  hand, 47, 148
  hip, 47
  knee, 47
rickets, 44, 141
Rigler's sign, 21, 125
rubella, 82

S
sacroiliac joint, seronegative arthritis, 48
sacroiliitis, 32, 33, 145
sail sign, 7
salivary diseases, 54
salt and pepper skull, 42, 141
sandostatin, 25
Saphena varix, 38
sarcoidosis, 110

sarcomatous metastases, 9
sausage digit, 48
scaphoid fracture, 139
sceroderma, 32
scintigraphy, 71, 72, 73–4
  tomographic, 74
sclerosing cholangitis, 29
sclerosis, 48, 152
sclerotic metastatic bone deposits, 139
scoliosis, 73
scrotal mass, 37–9
sebaceous cyst, 55
seizures, 58–9
Seldinger technique, 90
seminoma, 37, 137
seronegative arthropathy, 41
sigmoid volvulus, 20, 129
single photon emission computed tomography
      (SPECT), 93
Sjögren's syndrome, 54, 160
slipped capital femoral epiphysis (SCFE), 72–3,
      74–5, 170
slipped upper femoral epiphysis (SUFE), 170
Sloane-Kettering Level I–VI classification, 53
small bowel
  barium swallow, 89
  celiac disease, 32
  Crohn's disease, 31–2, 126
  malrotation, 167
  obstruction, 20, 126–7
  sceroderma, 32
small left colon, 67
smokers
  dysphagia, 17
  hemoptysis, 3
  Warthin's tumor, 54
sodium-iodide symporter chain, 95
soft tissue
  computed tomography, 90
  radiograph, 87
sphenoid sinus, 153
sphincterotomy, 22
spina bifida, 78, 79, 81
spine
  compression fracture, 146
  lumbar, radiography, 73, 114
  radiograph, 88, 142, 150
  rheumatoid arthritis, 47
  scoliosis, 73
  seronegative arthritis, 48
  vertebrae metastases, 144

spine *(Continued)*
 see also back pain
spleen, 91, 96
splenomegaly, 16
Staphylococcus, 73
 aureau, 50
stereotaxis, 13, 14
string sign of Kantor, 32, 126
stroke, 58, 91
subarachnoid hemorrhage, 57
subchondral cyst, 48
surfactant deficiency, 163
swan-neck deformity (fingers), 47
syndesmophytes, 41

T
Tc-labelled MAG-3, 63, 95
technetium, 93, 94–5
technetium antimony sulphide colloid, 96
technetium hepatoiminodiacetic acid (HIDA), 96
technetium HMPAO, 96
technetium human albumin nanocolloid, 95
technetium labelled heat denatured red blood
 cells, 96
technetium labelled sulphur colloid, 96
technetium methylene diphosphate, 95
technetium pertechnetate, 95
technetium tin colloid, 96
teratoma, 37
testis, 137
 ectropic/undescended, 38
 testicular microlithiasis, 38
 testicular neoplasm, 37
 testicular varicocele, 23, 137
 torsion, 37
thallium, 95
thoracic malignancy, 8
thrombosis, 91
 cerebral, 157
thyroglossal (duct) cyst, 54
thyroid
 hemithyroidectomy, 56
 metastases, 9
 nuclear medical imaging, 95
 thyroidectomy, 53
thyroid mass, 15, 53–4
 adenoma, 53
 anaplastic carcinoma, 54
 follicular carcinoma, 53–4

thyroid mass *(Continued)*
 hyperfunctioning nodule, 53
 papillary carcinoma, 53
thyroid nodule, 160
tibia, Paget's disease, 140
tibiotalar slant, 49
toddler's fracture, 73
tomogram, 148
tomographic scintigraphy (SPECT), 74
toxic megacolon, 33, 130
toxoplasmosis, 82
transabdominal ultrasound (TAS), 77
transient ischemic attack (TIA), 91
transient synovitis of the hip, 71
transvaginal ultrasound (TVUS), 77, 78
traumatic brain injury (TBI), 59–60
tuberculosis
 apical, 106
 colonic, 33
 miliary, 112
tumor imaging, 97
Turner's syndrome, 55

U
ulcerative colitis, 29, 31, 33, 41, 48, 128
ultrasound, 87, 91–2
 A mode echocardiography, 91
 abdominal, 91
 abdominal pain, 19, 26, 91
 abdominal/pelvic abscess, 24–5
 abortion, threatened, 77
 adenoma, 53
 amniocentesis, 81
 anencephaly, 78, 83
 bile duct stricture, 29
 bowel habit, altered, 35
 branchial cyst, 55
 breast abscess, 118
 breast carcinoma, 117
 breast mass, 13, 14
 Budd-Chiari syndrome, 91
 cardiac, 91–2
 chest pain, dyspnea or hemoptysis, 10
 cholangiocarcinoma, 29
 cirrhosis, 27
 common bile duct, 134
 cystic hygroma, 55
 development dysplasia of the hip (DDH),
 71, 166

ultrasound *(Continued)*
    Doppler, 29, 37, 38, 53, 82, 91, 116
    dysphagia, 15
    ectopic pregnancy, 24
    ectropic/undescended testicle, 38
    endoluminal, 15, 16
    endometriosis, 24
    esophageal varices, 16
    femoral artery aneurysm, 38
    fetal abnormality, screening for, 78–80
    fetal biometry, 80–1
    fetal death, 83
    fibroids (leiomyomata), 24
    first trimester, 77–8
    gallstones, 22
    groin mass, 37–9
    gynecological disease, 24–5
    hemangioma, 27
    hepatic cyst, 27
    hepatitis, 27
    hepatobiliary, 91
    hip dysplasia, 73
    hydatid disease, 28
    hydrocele, 37, 137
    hypertrophic pyloric stenosis, 168
    jaundice, 27, 91
    leukemia, 37
    lipoma, 55
    liver metastases, 28
    lymphadenopathy, 38
    lymphangioma, 55
    lymphoma, 37
    M mode echocardiography, 91
    molar (gestational trophoblastic disease), 78
    neck mass, 53, 55–6
    neurological disturbance, 91
    obstetric, 77–83
    ovarian cyst, torsion, 24
    pancreatic carcinoma, 29
    pancreatitis, 22
    pediatric radiology, 77–83, 91, 166
    pelvic, 91
    pelvic inflammatory disease, 25
    pseudoaneurysn, 38
    renal colic, 22
    renal malignancy, 23
    renal tract, 63, 64–5
    Saphena varix, 38
    sebaceous cyst, 55
    second trimester, 78–81

ultrasound *(Continued)*
    seminoma, 37, 137
    septic arthritis, 71
    stroke, 91
    teratoma, 37
    testes, 37, 137
    third trimester, 81–3
    thrombosis, 91
    thyroglossal (duct) cyst, 54
    thyroid mass, 15
    thyroid nodule, 160
    transabdominal (TAS), 25, 77
    transient synovitis of the hip, 71
    transvaginal (TVUS), 25, 77, 78
    ulcerative colitis, 33
    urinary tract infection, 23, 65
    varicocele, 37, 137
    venous insufficiency, 91
umbilical artery Doppler, 82
urinary tract infection (UTI), 23
    childhood, 63–5
    lower, 63
    obstructive uropathies, 63
    upper, 63
urography, 89–90, 136
urological diseases, 22–3
    fetal obstructive uropathies, 80
uterine mass, 81, 82
uterus, 91

V
VACTERL, 68
Valsalva maneuver, 37
varicocele, 37, 137
vena cava, 91
ventilation-perfusion (VQ) scan, 94–5
    chest pain, dyspnea or hemoptysis, 3, 10
    mismatch, 7, 94
    pulmonary embolus, 7, 104
ventricular failure, 3–4
ventriculomegaly, 79
vesico-uretic reflux (VUR), 63, 64, 168
vipoma, 97
vitamin D deficiency, 44
voiding cystourethrogram (VCUG),
    63, 65, 168
volvulus, 20, 70, 167
    cecal, 20
    sigmoid, 20, 129
voxel, 90

W
Warthin's tumor, 54
water, computed tomography, 90
Westermark sign, 7
Whipple's disease, 41, 48
white cell imaging, 96
white matter diseases, 58

X
X-rays, 87
  see also abdominal X-ray (AXR); chest X-ray
    (CXR); radiograph
xenon, 95